Supermodels'
diet
secrets

simple strategies
for staying slim
from the world's
top models

Victoria Nixon

PIATKUS

Copyright © 2004 by Victoria Nixon

First published in 2004 by
Piatkus Books Ltd
5 Windmill Street
London W1T 2JA

e-mail: info@piatkus.co.uk

The opinions and advice expressed in this book are intended as a guide only. Neither the publisher nor the author is engaged in rendering professional advice or services to the individual reader. If you have a medical condition or are pregnant, the diet described in this book should not be followed without first consulting your doctor. The publisher and author accept no responsibility for any injury or loss sustained as a result of using this book.

The moral right of the author has been asserted

A catalogue record for this book is available from the British Library

ISBN 0 7499 2517 5

Edited by Jan Cutler

This book has been printed on paper manufactured with respect for the environment using wood from managed sustainable resources

Data manipulation by Phoenix Photosetting, Chatham, Kent
Printed and bound in Great Britain by Mackays Ltd, Chatham, Kent

Contents

Acknowledgements

Thank you to the models who gave their insights and time so generously, and to my ace editor Alice Davis, who stayed cool when I developed severe writer's block while writing about constipation and high-protein diets.

A big hug to Paula for managing the deli superbly while I was working on the book, and for being astute enough never to ask, 'How's the book coming along then?', especially during the above crisis.

And megathanks to Michael who, for some unfathomable reason, always makes me feel happy and makes all things possible.

Introduction

I know, I know – who in her right mind would write a book about models and food? Were two subjects ever so diametrically opposed, so mutually exclusive, so perfectly honed to be the bony butt of endless 'grissini stick' guffaws?

Slender girls in the world of fashion – it's long been a delicate, sensitive issue: the ever-vigilant press constantly updating us on the current thigh measurement of every young girl to grace the catwalk. Yet, contrary to popular belief, the top girls – the supermodels – don't stay slim because they have a smack habit, live on champagne and cigarettes or have 'disorders'. They're actually hard-working career girls who constantly travel the world alone, booked months ahead for blindingly expensive advertising campaigns and achingly close-up magazine covers. It's a life of go, show and glow, where airbrushing is not an option.

Unlike their iconic Hollywood sisters, supermodels do not have nutritionists or personal chefs on their payroll. Not for them the divadom of employing diet coaches, who earn their crusts by offering up the latest snippet on carb reduction in the eternal, faddy search for bodily perfection.

Supermodels don't do diets. In fact most of them have never dieted in their lives. What they use are simple skills and instantly workable strategies that don't cost a bean but keep their wise owners slim and healthy for the duration of their careers and long after they retire. Truthfully, when did you last see a photograph of a fat former top model? Cindy Crawford, Jerry Hall, Marie Helvin, Twiggy, Lauren Hutton *et al.* still possess the figures that made them famous and continue to look great in their late thirties, forties, fifties and beyond in a world where some television presenters' girths appear to expand the minute their careers constrict.

The fact is the majority of supermodels love food with a satiable passion, and they're likely to laugh in your face – or punch it – if you ever doubt their healthy eating habits. And no, they're not automatically gifted with some miraculous genetic template for weight control that eludes other women and means they never have to watch their weight. Sophie Dahl worked hard to shed those famous pounds, and Jodie Kidd made 'heroin chic' très un-chic when she made a determined effort to increase her weight.

The crucial difference between models and many other women is that models are able to sustain a consistent weight for the long term, which they do in order to make a living, and not because they have a family wedding, a party or a forthcoming holiday to get in shape for. It is this learned ability to stay the course that is the key to keeping a slim figure for life.

Models incorporate realistic strategies and a wealth of professional trade skills into their daily routine until it becomes second nature. They use wisdom, not waffle, to retrain their old habits. Overeating, eating rubbish and binge eating are easier to overcome with the right tools – and you don't have to put your life on hold to achieve success.

You don't need to go to a place to be weighed and applauded for getting it right, as models well know. You don't need group leaders or diet sheets to control your food intake. You can stay in shape without ever spending money on meal replacements and slimming products, or staying at home concocting miserable meals that taste like blotting paper. Nor do you need the dangerous diets where you stuff yourself full of protein and saturated fats for extended periods of time. We already know that they give you halitosis, but what about kidney damage, heart disease, osteoporosis, bowel cancer and severe depression? We won't know how safe the Atkins type of diet is for years.

Ah, those diet books – are there any readers left out there who still need to be informed that a pizza makes you fatter than an apple? Then it's the carbs versus fats debate: which works best, which produces the quickest results? Most diet books focus on one or the other. How many calories does a muffin have compared with a croissant or an old sock?.... Is there more fat in a sausage roll or a hot dog? ... Still awake? If I were Mogadon I'd sue most diet books for theft of patent. Yet diet books and cookery books abound. How to get thin, how to get fat; it's either too hard to swallow or culled from the school of the absolutely bloomin' obvious.

Come on, we've all realised by now that a one-dimensional diet is boring, time-consuming and leaves you unsupported when it stops. Inevitably, you regain the weight, and then you feel a failure, when actually it's the diet that has failed you! We all know we should eat only in direct proportion to what we can burn off – but staying slim is more than the sum of these parts. Men overeat when they're part of a social gathering. Women mostly overeat alone. It's a multi-faceted emotional conundrum of the complex female psyche, and not simply a question of jiggling and juggling carbs, proteins, sugar and fats.

In short, the quick fix doesn't work for women – ever! Let's finally get real. The only way to lose weight for good is never to go on a diet again! Top models know it's the long-term results that count. It's changing the tiny things in your daily life that lead to the really big differences. What you weigh and how you look in ten years' time is not determined by what you do in the next ten hours, days or weeks, but by what you do *consistently* for the next ten years. Successful models (a) balance what they eat; (b) eat food they really enjoy; and (c) know when to stop, and these are the very skills the slimming world and the less scrupulous elements of the food industry don't want you to master, but more of that later.

Modelling appears to be a glamorous life, but it can be exhausting and lonely: finding your way around foreign countries, checking into hotels, locating studios, and working with a bunch of strangers isn't that much fun without a chaperone, let alone an entourage. As Kate Moss says, you need to be strong to survive it. My shameless love of good food emerged during my modelling years on the international circuit. That succulent pastrami on rye in New York; my favourite cheese shop in the Rue de

Tocqueville in Paris; the aroma therapy of my local coffee bar in Milan ... Oh God, I could go on and on ... made the global fashion merry-go-round infinitely more palatable.

Then came an epiphanic moment when I *absolutely* got the point about eating good food. I don't mean poring over long menus in flashy restaurants, but the pure and complete realisation that eating is not always about simply refuelling your body, stuffing your face, or constantly counting calories, but about discovering the sublime sensuality of great and diverse tastes.

So I opened my own deli in London and I now have hundreds of irresistible smells, visual treats, tastes and textures under one roof. Take it from me, eating well does not restrict you – it frees you – from guilt, denial and deprivation. I can prove it: after 12 years of deli life I'm still the same dress size as in the good old modelling days – and Gym and I have never been close friends.

An absolute love of good food is a joyous thing but no more joyous than a healthy, slim body. For this book I have marinated my experiences as a model and subsequent deli owner with the skills and tips so generously donated by the beautiful and gracious top models kind enough to be interviewed.

I think we've invented a refreshing recipe for genuine long-term slimming success that's guaranteed to work. We want you to try it. Why? Because you're worth it.

Part One
Head Start

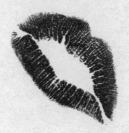

'How you think is always more important than what you eat because the right thoughts will guide you towards food that is nourishing and healthy.'

Catherine Hurley
*From Medical student (St Hilda's, Oxford)
to supermodel
Campaigns: Lacoste, Max Factor, Vogue & Elle
regular*

1

Train your brain to listen to your body

If dieting really worked, we'd only have to do it once. Diets fail because our minds are constantly fighting our bodies. And the diet industry constantly tries to seduce us with their short-term solutions, without giving a damn about the impact their wares have on our physical and mental well-being. They don't care why we want to diet in the first place. They choose to focus on goal weights and calorie- and carbohydrate-counting regimes, which they know will ensure we return for more punishment when our willpower caves in. So we're bombarded with more recipes we'll never have time to make, more last-minute shopping for the ridiculous meals we're allowed to eat, and more promises of 'a new body in two weeks' so that we can fit into our party frocks. Don't the scientists, and lifestyle gurusomes who invent these diets, realise that women have busy, real lives and that a successful, healthy diet is more about small lifestyle changes than simply a matter of science and chemistry?

Women are perverse creatures: constantly going to extremes, walking the tightrope between goodness and harm, and awash with contradictions as we try to keep our balance in life. We eat organic then scoff cheap chocolate; go to a yoga class then light a cigarette, drink more vodka than we should because it's 'pure' and enjoy sunbathing for two weeks in Spain, then hit expensive anti-wrinkle creams for the rest of the year. We work hard, run just to keep up, buy more and more designer goods to make us happy, and compete to be the best-looking trader on the floor, the thinnest mum on the school run, the shapeliest belle of the ball, the comeliest girl on the catwalk. We constantly strive for unattainable standards of beauty. It's not surprising that looking great often appears to be a damage-limitation exercise for life.

The right mental approach to the way you look

Like it or not, how we look affects how other people treat us, and how other people treat us affects the way we lead our lives. Yet a thin body is no guarantee of happiness and it's important to get beyond the idea that life is all about the shape of our thighs. When we constantly try to airbrush our reality, it gets in the way of our real achievements.

What's the right shape anyway? It's dangerous to distort a body to conform to a fashionable shape of the moment if it is not inclined to do so. Not everyone is meant to be whippet thin – thank goodness. Women tend to think you can't be too thin, but you can. A top fashion designer may endorse the super-thin waifs who trail down the catwalks sporting his bizarre, unwearable creations as the perfect coat-hangers, but who wants to be compared to a piece of wire?

> *While it has long been held that a successful couture model requires the dimensions of a coat-hanger, the supermodels proved the body fascists wrong by carrying the collections with total aplomb. A stick-thin arm dangling out of a £20,000 gown is far less enticing than a set of fleshy curves — all hail the new womanly shape.*
>
> **Laura Craik, Fashion Editor,**
> **Evening Standard, London**

A woman checks herself in a mirror an average of five times a day, but she tends to focus on her worst features and imperfections rather than appraise the whole picture. Former top model Cameron Diaz, now one of the highest paid actress in Hollywood, would be the first to tell you she has problem skin and is constantly prone to spots. Yet what *we* see are expressive eyes and a beguiling smile. Her entire personality shines through her less-than-perfect complexion.

> *All women have insecurities about their body and I'm no different, even though I'm used to*

the camera. My feelings about my body change from day to day. Some mornings I wake up and feel confident, but sometimes I have an off day so I'll do things to make myself feel better, such as going for a massage or meeting up with girl-friends for a glass of wine.'

Laura Bailey

Ask any model and she'll tell you there's nothing more deflating than walking into a model-casting session where you perceive all the other waiting girls to be infinitely more attractive than yourself – and then having your looks dissected by clients as though you're a contender at Crufts.

During my modelling days, I remember sitting in a room while clients discussed my portfolio of work photographs. 'She'd be great for the job if it wasn't for *that*,' they all said in unison, pointing to a picture in the folio and assessing the real-life version with cold, narrow eyes. What...? Nose hair? Bunions? Filthy fingernails? Saggy kneecaps? Entire head and body? What...? Another job rejection, and I never did find out what *that* was. Just as well. Next casting!

'When you don't really look like anyone else, have a nose that's not going to go away and don't really develop breasts, it's important to learn to accept your body the way it is. It's not to do with weight or body image but I had to come to terms with the features I was given. It's amazing because now they've been celebrated.'

Erin O'Connor

Are you truly ready for change?

Our body image sometimes influences everything in our lives. 'If only I could change my weight I'd be happier/more successful/have fewer problems/be a better person ...' But, when you try to change your eating patterns, if you start with very low self-esteem related to the way you look, you simply won't last long.

Your sense of self is based on past experiences, successes and failures, other people's opinions and your own reactions to all of these. Your own beliefs may have an unduly negative influence over the way you deal with food. It's impossible to get slim until you are 'slim' in your mind, then your body will automatically follow.

If you try to do it the other way round, with the sole emphasis on the food aspect, you may lose weight short term, but sooner or later it will all come back; the weight goes – the problem stays.

We all have the power to change the way we view ourselves and improve our appearance, but the correct mental approach is vital. First, it's important to believe firmly that you can control your weight rather than it controlling you, and this means addressing some important issues. If you've lost weight in the past and then put it all back on, ask yourself why. Do you secretly enjoy the challenge and attention you get from permanently going on and off diets? Will becoming more attractive and healthy mean endless effort with your appearance, rather than the safety and comfort of your familiar old tracksuit?

Have you seriously thought through the implications of being fitter and therefore more attractive for life? This is not simply knocking off a few pounds for the summer but a psychological change to eat well permanently. It means you'll have more energy, fewer colds, glossier hair, younger-looking skin, clearer eyes and a sharper mind.

This change may give you more power and attention, which turns the spotlight on you and, in turn, may upset other people. Perhaps you feel you aren't worth the care and effort and that a change may deprive you of the foods you love. Think of all the areas where you could possibly sabotage yourself before you embark on this different approach to eating.

Many models have experienced a glitch in their attempt to attain their correct body image, often because they listened to too many diverse opinions from other people. When they finally got it right, they were able to step back, analyse, and then use it as part of their motivation.

> 'At the beginning of my career I was told to have breast implants and maybe shave my nose down, by people who didn't really understand or were too afraid to really accept me as I was.'
>
> Erin O'Connor

Recognising and accepting your setbacks may mean listing the times you've tried to lose weight in your life and why you went off track. You could find it was the same situation playing itself over and over again.

Life can only be understood backwards, but it must be

lived forwards. You can't change what happened to you in the past but you can use past mistakes to learn how to cope in the same situation in the future.

Think about the weight that suited you best in your life, when you felt and looked great. Aim to be that weight again. Get used to feeling comfortable about the idea of becoming that weight again. If you're not sure when you looked your best, ask a friend, a family member or a partner. You might be surprised by their answer.

> *The photographer Richard Avedon once told me, "Cindy, you don't look good when you're very thin, your face gets too skinny." So I used that as an excuse to be the weight that suits me rather than what is fashionable.'*
>
> **Cindy Crawford**

As you change weight, visualise yourself slim and attractive in the clothes you want to wear, and picture how other people will react to you at your new weight. Concentrate on the feelings these thoughts evoke, and you will send a message to your brain that will affect your energy levels, motivation and metabolism.

These changes cause physical sensations, which in turn affect your thoughts and emotions. It's a positive feedback system. We become not only what we eat but what we think as well.

Don't, however, think of this different approach to your eating pattern as yet another 'diet'. The very word conjures up deprivation and denial, which is sad because the Ancient

Greek word *diata*, from which we get the word diet, simply meant 'way of life'. Think of this as your new way of life.

Beyond being slim

Before we move on from the area of body image, I need to say one thing: if you secretly bought this book because you thought it might be an endorsement for very thin women, you'll be disappointed. The fashion business is constantly blamed for encouraging young, impressionable girls to lose weight, but most of the supermodels they wish to emulate don't diet and have never dieted. Sometimes a young girl's body goes through a natural phase of being very thin before it takes on a womanly shape. Often the models who were naturally skinny in their teens didn't enjoy their shape either.

The business about my weight was very upsetting, but I know that I never had a problem. Now I'm still long and bony but I've put on two stone and have breasts. I love being this size and feel more like a woman now. I finally feel sexy. I grew into my body when I was 22 and that's when I grew up.'

Jodie Kidd

Eating disorders, such as anorexia nervosa, bulimia nervosa and serious forms of binge-eating disorder, are usually symptoms of deep emotional distress, although they may have started as a diet that then went too far. Young girls aged around 12–25 are the most at risk of anorexia nervosa. Bulimia nervosa and binge-eating disorder tends to affect older women, although these conditions can occur at any age. They also affect men, although it's much less common.

Often people with anorexia nervosa have experienced pressure from their peer groups and parents to be ultra competitive and achieve well. Their mantra is 'If I can stick to my special (unhealthy) diet I'll feel successful, be in control, and be popular.'

Although many recover from anorexia, about half never fully recover, and about a third will be seriously affected by it throughout their life.

'I think teachers and schools could do much more to understand this problem. I'm very aware of the responsibility I have to the models I represent and the image they represent to young girls who are living in a world that's increasingly obsessed with body image.'

Sarah Doukas
Storm Model Agency, representing
Kate Moss, Elle Macpherson,
Sophie Dahl, Liberty Ross

Stomach or head hunger?
....

Putting food in our mouths is primal and comforting. But what really makes us eat? Is it because we're hungry, because we like the look of something, because we mark time at certain points of the day, or because it brings a moment's relief in our fast-moving world? In other words, is it genuine hunger or an emotional need? Sure, gut-wrenching physical hunger gives us our basic drive to eat, but eating can also be suppressed by emotion or by consciously defying our instinctive drive to eat – as in strict dieting or in eating disorders.

Most of us eat more than our bodies need because food is so abundant that eating purely for hunger is rare rather than a given. Food today is cleverly advertised, seductively packaged, quickly prepared, confusingly labelled and mega-sized. Because it's so accessible, it's only too easy to use it to cope with life's ups and downs.

We eat mindlessly – in front of the telly, behind our desks, wrapped around a steering wheel. We used to hunt and dig for food and appreciate what we found, but now we drive to supermarkets, and heat and serve.

What and why we eat is influenced by learned automatic responses and habits, which have nothing to do with true physical hunger. When we find it hard to express anger or deal with insecure feelings, food is a useful means of stuffing all that emotion back down. The most common reason for overeating is to attempt to change the way we feel. I remember once using overeating to cope with a seemingly hopeless situation when I was an ingénue model. Booked for a swimwear shoot on a tropical island, with a well-known photographer and another model from my agency, I knew the photographer and model were having a secret affair. The photographer's wife was also a model with the same agency – and my best friend. Would I be seen as an enabler if the affair leaked out? What to do?

As the trip got nearer and nearer, I found myself eating more and more until I was cancelled for the job. What a relief – I didn't have to disappoint my agency by turning down the trip in the first place, or tell the truth to my friend. Forcing my body to be too fat for the job seemed less painful than confronting the real issues.

What I hadn't reckoned on was how uncomfortable, unhappy and unfit I felt carrying around all those extra pounds. But it was a hell of a lot more pleasure piling them on than taking them off.

From then on, I learned to say 'No' firmly and effectively and made myself some rules that kept me slim for the rest of my career. I feel lucky that I recognised the influence emotional thinking has on the body – that it's not simply a question of calories, fats, exercise and willpower.

'Modelling has taught me to stand up for myself. I've become much more assertive when choosing my modelling jobs and defend my interests. I've also become more outspoken and have learned to say "No" with grace, in a way that doesn't upset people, which I wasn't very good at before.'

Catherine Hurley

2

Breaking old habits

The food we prefer, and all our eating patterns, are formed in childhood, when food was often used as a bartering tool, reward or punishment. It's important to realise that how we were brought up strongly influences our relationship with food in later life.

Some of us were given too many trashy snacks rather than fruit or yoghurt, which left us with an ultra-sweet tooth. Others were told about all the starving children who would be happy to have their food, when they struggled to clear their plates. And some had mothers who, themselves, had neurotic, unhealthy relationships with food.

Maybe you come from a family where seconds or even thirds were considered a polite compliment to your mother's cooking, and when the message came through that you were full, you simply ignored it, and demolished whatever remained on your plate.

TIP From now on always leave something on your plate – even if it's just one bean. This sends a message to your mind that you're breaking old patterns of eating.

Remember: hunger and appetite are not the same – hunger is a nagging sensation that kick-starts constant thoughts of food and reminds us that our bodies want to eat; appetite is the tendency to eat. After the main course you may not feel hungry but you still have a tendency to eat. *Hunger* is how you feel, but *appetite* is how much you eat.

Only *you* can *now* decide what to put into your mouth, and that decision starts in your head. It's important that you don't always blame circumstances for your behaviour and that you take full responsibility for your habits. The key is to think *why* you want to eat in a given situation; to make eating a conscious action rather than a continuing habit – to make food your friend, rather than your enemy.

TIP Whenever you're not enjoying what you're eating – stop. Your body is telling you it's not right for you now and it doesn't need it.

How you think is always more important than what you eat, because the right thoughts will guide you towards nourishing food. Saying you won't eat much today because you want to lose weight will find you starving hungry. But if you say you're going to eat sensibly today, starting with a good breakfast, your body will respond by giving you the energy to carry you through.

Kicking the fast-food habit
· ·

Your body is the greatest machine on earth, and when you eat proper food it functions like a well-oiled engine; it responds to healthy eating because it's designed to do so. The problems arise when you stuff it full of junk. Most of the food that models eat is recognisable from its natural origins. Proper, real food is freshly picked, gathered, milked, hunted or fished, and the further food strays from this basis, the unhealthier and the more confusing it can become for your body to cope with.

Apart from being nutritionally deficient, processed foods make you hungrier than you actually are. Big portions are also cheap to produce, and manufacturers realise we think with our eyes and get seduced by quantity, not quality. It's worth noting that a standard bag of crisps in the UK is now double the weight it used to be. So fast food is the lazy person's dream – you hardly have to chew it, let alone prepare it.

When we eat healthy food it produces the feelgood brain chemicals dopamine and serotonin (from specific amino acids contained in the proteins we eat), which help us to listen directly to our bodies. Dopamine is similar to adren-aline and affects how we move, our emotional responses and our ability to experience pleasure and pain. But it is serotonin that is the brain's primary good mood chemical and is responsible for feelings of comfort, satisfaction, contentment, happiness, relaxation and optimism.

TIP Eat well and you won't have the desire to eat to feel good. You'll eat only because you're hungry – and when you're really hungry food tastes great, especially fresh, simple, healthy food.

Many women are deficient in serotonin, and low levels are associated with food cravings and depression. Research shows that *all* obese women are deficient in serotonin. So, it's absolutely vital to provide your body with the nutrients necessary to produce adequate serotonin.

This essential brain chemical is mainly produced in the morning, and eating a healthy breakfast will balance your brain so that you'll want to eat the right amount of healthier foods during the day. If you skip breakfast or eat an imbalance of nutrients for the rest of the day, it'll take all the willpower you possess to keep away from junk food.

When your brain is out of chemical balance, you'll always crave unhealthy food , and if you're unhappy you'll want foods that give you a momentary lift. Unfortunately, they'll then leave you depleted and even more unhappy. If you're aware you're 'junking out' too often, start by surrounding yourself only with healthier foods, and initially avoid all contact with junk food. Just seeing or smelling it can trigger emotional hunger, even though your body doesn't want or need it. Avoiding junk is much easier when you're producing adequate brain chemicals, and when you feel fitter you can eat fast food occasionally without doing damage to your system.

> **TIP** After about nine days of feeding your brain cells well in the mornings, your tastes begin to change automatically – and healthy food starts to taste fantastic.

Try not to miss a meal ever when you change from junk food to healthier food, and don't deprive yourself. Eat as much as your body wants, to begin with. Soon it will take no willpower whatsoever and you'll want to eat only the amount of food your body needs and can digest.

Why models use flexible restraint

The very nature of a model's work means she must maintain a steady weight for her entire career. Using 'flexible restraint' allows her to follow a healthy-eating routine most of the time, but sometimes include favourite comfort foods or have an exotic meal out, as opposed to 'rigid restraint', which involves strict unbending dietary rules.

Most models prefer to use the 80/20 ratio, eating healthy, real food for 80 per cent per cent of the time and using the remaining 20 per cent for treats.

Flexible restraint greatly reduces the risk of 'all or nothing' thinking, relapsing and bingeing. It helps you to be satisfied with small amounts of your favourite foods, knowing you can eat them again sometimes, rather than a particular occasion being your 'last chance'. It's a sign that you're in control of your food choices and your weight, rather than them controlling you.

Research shows us that flexible restraint works brilliantly for long-term weight control, whether you're maintaining a healthy weight or trying to lose some. Those who slimmed successfully in recent tests developed a personal and flexible approach to eating, while those who failed generally opted for rigid plans.

> ### Food for thought
> Why is it that people on diets spend all their time thinking about food – except when they're actually eating? Then they try not to notice what's happening.

The binge factor

We all over-indulge sometimes – even supermodels. Which one of us hasn't scoffed an entire packet of HobNobs when we've been really down? Oh, probably a few lifestyle guru-somes, living their perfect, over-disciplined lives – but do we want to know them? Not in this life thanks.

Yet over-indulging with food, and a 'binge', can mean different things to different people. A serious binge has *both* the following characteristics:

1. Eating much more fattening food than you would normally eat within a short period of time.

2. Feeling out of control during the eating period. It's this feeling of 'lack of control' along with guilt and remorse after the binge that really distinguishes a binge from overeating.

Some of us may have a true binge without it being a real problem, whereas others binge frequently, to the extent that it seriously affects their lives. Many doctors believe that, as with other serious eating disorders, cognitive behavioural therapy is the most helpful way to tackle the problem, as it focuses on the cause rather than the food.

TIP Think about what would make you particularly happy. Another chocolate bar that will last a few minutes, or a fantastic body that will last a lifetime?

Binge thinking

Eating when you're not hungry doesn't just happen, even though it might feel like it does. It's the end result of a chain of events that have several triggers. Below are the most common triggers listed under two headings: environmental and emotional, and it is worth ticking the ones that could apply to you.

ENVIRONMENTAL	EMOTIONAL
Confusing hunger with thirst	Boredom or loneliness
Premenstrual symptoms	Exhaustion or anxiety
Not having healthy foods at hand	Feeling deprived of food
Missing a meal	Anger or depression
Preparing food	Feeling deserving of reward
Drinking alcohol	Guilt about overeating
Too much spare time	Feeling unattractive
The smell of food	Relationship problems
Food advertisements and recipes	Sadness, hopelessness
Shopping when hungry	Spiritual emptiness
TV food programmes	Feeling unfulfilled

Once you know what your triggers are, you can learn to respond to them in a different way. Next time you have an urge to overeat, ask yourself, 'When did I last eat? Why do I want to eat when my last meal was so recent and I don't feel any "stomach hunger"?'

This questioning approach allows you time to identify your triggers, choose whether to eat or not and, if you do, to choose healthy food you really enjoy. A craving rarely lasts longer than 15 or 20 minutes so you need to distract yourself. Clean your teeth, then do something you enjoy – phone or visit a friend, go for a walk, have a relaxing bath.

Never beat yourself up if you get off track. It isn't a problem in itself, but how you react to it. One slip-up doesn't mean you've undone all your hard work. Put it behind you, get back on track and learn from it.

Remember that what you weigh and how you look in ten years' time is not determined by what you do in the next ten hours, days or weeks, but by what you do *consistently* for the next ten years.

> **TIP** Instead of heading straight to the fridge or drinks cupboard for a numbing blast when you get home from work, have a bath or shower to wash away the stress of the day. You'll feel much more relaxed to taste and enjoy your drink and food.

Anti-binge tactics

The following will help you avoid the circumstances which may make you feel you need to overeat:

- Identify and isolate your trigger food.

- Don't keep trigger foods in the house; sooner or later you'll eat them.

- Don't give yourself treats that may be your trigger foods.

- Realise it's the initial taste of food, salty or sweet, that promotes the craving.

- Never go shopping on an empty stomach.

- Use a displacement activity when you feel the desire to binge.

- Don't eat while watching telly, reading a magazine or talking on the phone.

- Never miss a meal. You'll end up eating too much too quickly and then feel guilty.

- Eat something every three hours, even if it's just a piece of fruit.

- If you lapse, don't beat yourself up. It could cause you to carry on.

- Remember: it's a long-term project to be healthy for the rest of your life.

- Have cosy, substitute comfort foods in your cupboards.

- When eating out, have a non-trigger healthy snack before leaving home.

Auto-suggestion

Try this idea if there is a consistent binge food you want out of your life. Think of a food you hate. Now, vividly recall how much you hate it – it's awful smell and taste. As you do this, push your thumb into the centre of the palm of your hand. Do this at least five times, each time vividly recalling how much you hate that food. Stop and relax. Now think about your binge food and push your thumb into the centre of the palm of your hand, again five times. Repeat this process every time you feel compelled to binge.

All snacked out

Models are only too aware that the advertising industry is full of trickery – from airbrushing all conceivable character from their photographed faces to sell cosmetics, to cunningly editing a naive blonde giving oral pleasure to a chocolate log (okay, I confess to being the flaky talent in that commercial; but, hey, a girl had to make a living).

One of the oldest ever advertising wheezes is to associate chocolate bars with slogans that lead us to believe we can't get through the day without the product. Because of this strong association, it's a good idea to replace the word 'snack' with another word that automatically triggers more healthy choices in your mind than 'pop in your gob' crisps, chocolates and sweets. You'll find yourself quickly improving your 'crap consumption' if you break up your day with 'energisers' rather than 'snacks'.

How healthy is your relationship with food?

Which of the following statements relate to you? Add up the number given in brackets to give your total score. Do you:

1. Leave home in the morning without having breakfast? (4)

2. Choose fattening food even when you know what to eat to be slim? (4)

3. Always feel guilty after eating chocolate, crisps or biscuits? (2)

4. Feel you need an edible treat to cheer you up if you're miserable? (3)

5. Need something sweet to get you through the afternoon at work? (1)

6. Have clothes for when you're heavier and others for when you're slimmer? (3)

7. Eat more chocolate or ice cream when you're on your own? (3)

8. Sometimes go right through the afternoon without eating? (3)

9. Find it difficult to stop once you've started eating sweets or snacks? (4)

10. Not like to eat in front of people you don't know? (2)

11. Wish you were slimmer? (1)

12. Feel you can eat chocolate if you're with a friend who's eating it? (3)

13. Sometimes eat something before going out to dinner so it looks like you've got a smaller appetite later? (5)

14. Always clear your plate and always have dessert even if you're full? (4)

15. Admit you're heavier now than five years ago, even though you're always dieting? (3)

16. Constantly try new diets but never stick to them for more than a few weeks? (3)

17. Never eat three or more portions of vegetables and fruit a day? (3)

18. Sometimes eat a whole meal without really tasting it? (4)

19. Always buy prepared meals marked low fat or low calorie? (2)

20. Know you should exercise but really can't be bothered? (4)

IF YOU SCORED 10 OR LESS: no worries. You probably only have a few pounds to lose, if at all, and know exactly what you need to do to lose them. You don't have any major psychological problems with food.

IF YOU SCORED 11–25: you might be a bit overweight and you eat out of habit when you're bored or under stress. Your main problem is using food to take your mind off other problems rather than for giving you the nutrients you need, or for pleasure. Training your mind to think differently about food can easily change that.

IF YOU SCORED 26–40: you probably have an emotional relationship with food and dieting, which stops you from eating sensibly and reaching your ideal weight easily. Your weight itself is unlikely to be a major problem, but you'd be happier if you were in control of your weight. This is the time to change your attitude towards food for good.

IF YOU SCORED 41–60: your weight and eating is a big issue for you. You are probably a yo-yo dieter – constantly going on and coming off diets – and suffer from mood swings, tiredness, irritability and very low self-esteem. This is all about to change. This should be the last 'diet' you ever follow.

3

Exploding a few myths

At some point in their lives, all models realise that simply watching what they eat isn't, in itself, going to do it for them. It only all starts coming together when they develop an ongoing awareness, an ability to define successfully what works and what doesn't in the long-term objective of staying slim.

It takes common sense, knowledge of the true facts and a canny mental approach to sift through the mounds of misleading nutritional nonsense and separate it from the genuinely useful skills that ensure a life-long healthy attitude to eating. In this section we look at the ways you can protect yourself from the pitfalls, old wives' tales and convenient excuses that may sabotage your progress – and inject some smart strategies and model tricks into your life to stay ahead of the game.

The truth about 'fat' attitudes

· ·

The myths about weight loss and diets are endless and very dangerous – undermining the determination and motivation of women who simply wish to know the real facts about becoming fit, healthy and slim.

MYTH: 'All my family are obese, so it's in my genes and I can't do anything about it.'

TRUTH: Your genes play a minor role compared to a mutual preference for high-fat foods and low levels of spontaneous physical activity. Families usually share the same diet, lifestyle and cultural influences, and these habits tend to persist into later life.

MYTH: 'I have a thyroid problem which makes me fat.'

TRUTH: It's actually quite rare for medical conditions to cause obesity directly. Thyroid disease resulting in an underactive thyroid, which slows the metabolic rate, is not an important cause of obesity.

MYTH: 'She can eat what she likes and never gains weight, because she has a high metabolic rate.'

TRUTH: Actually slim people have lower resting metabolic rates than obese people because their vital organs are smaller and need fewer calories to function. In tests, all subjects gained weight at the same rate. The truth is that some people are more spontaneously active than others – they move, fidget, twitch or change position more often.

Is detoxing worth the effort?

The idea behind detoxing is that poisons from unhealthy food and polluted air build up in our tissues and put a strain on our organs, especially those involved with excreting waste, such as the liver. Detox enthusiasts believe that taking a break from your usual diet helps to reduce your toxin levels. They claim that this can be done by fasting, eating special foods and using products, such as the herbal remedy milk thistle, which aids liver function, that aim to support the body's eliminatory processes.

The main problem with cold-turkey detoxing is the side effects. Carol Vorderman warns that during the first week of her 28-day detox, you can expect pounding headaches, flatulence, sugar and caffeine cravings, and exhaustion. Enthusiasts say these are symptoms of a 'healing crisis' or signs of toxins leaving the body. Strewth! Surely it's easier to eat fairly sensibly most of the time instead. Your body's designed to rid itself of unwanted toxins without a detoxification programme. Your heart doesn't stop beating because it needs a rest. And how can anyone with a busy life stick to a rigid plan for 28 days and be sick as a dog for a week?

'I don't detox because I don't believe it's necessary if you eat well. I start the day with hot water with ginger or mint, and take aloe vera and milk thistle, and that sets me up for the day. I can't imagine detoxing for weeks on end.

*Having done your penance, you'd just want to go
mad and undo all the good.'*
Catherine Hurley

Detoxing's central theme is initially fasting on fresh
juices and making healthy little 'snacks' to pop in the fridge
to nibble on later. Fine, if you have a few spare hours to get
out the juicer, cut, peel and slice, and create endless fun
fruit and vegetable cocktails. But I find juicing a bit like
going to the gym: very worthy but it takes time and effort,
there's too much equipment, a lot of cleaning up afterwards
and sooner or later the gimmick wears off. You can also
have too much of a good thing. Juices made purely from
green-leafed vegetables are so strong they can cause nausea
and headaches and should be diluted with water or fruit
juice and sipped very slowly.

If you feel sluggish or out of sorts, simply increase your
still water intake from the moment you get up in the
morning all through the day, cut out rubbish food and
empty calories from your diet, elbow caffeine and alcohol,
and make green vegetables and salads the central part of
each meal outside of breakfast until you feel perkier. Eating
vegetables whole gives you the benefit of fibre that juicing
doesn't.

*'I don't have the time or inclination to go to some
place and be pampered and cleaned out, but if
it makes some people happy, why not?'*
India Hicks

If you have a spare, non-active weekend and you've been working or playing hard, it's not a bad idea to cleanse your system gently. Short-term detoxing may not do you any harm, but to do it for a month? It's the same old story – deprive yourself now and you'll want to make up for it later.

Allergic to the truth
....

Wheat-free, dairy-free, fat-free, carb-free – an incredible 40 per cent of women in the UK have banned specific foods from their daily diets over the past five years, believing they have some kind of food allergy or intolerance. Meanwhile ultra-hip nutritionists preach the gospel of health by banning virtually every edible food, when actually what they're doing is encouraging neurotic behaviour and inviting illness, even anorexia.

The most frightening aspect of faddy 'health' diets is the fine line between the anorexic, who painstakingly cuts her peas in four, and the 'careful' eater who picks the bread-crumbs off her veal scaloppini because she's wheat intolerant or on a low-carb 'health and energy' diet. Also scary is the number of women who assume an intolerance without getting their symptoms checked out by a health professional. It's worth noting that a significant number of doctors believe women are putting themselves at risk by cutting out important nutrients without medical or nutritional advice.

Among the health risks are malnutrition, nutrient deficiency, osteoporosis and immune problems. The common culprits of suspected food intolerances are wheat and dairy, but the Atkins type of diet has also contributed to women avoiding whole food groups, such as carbohydrates.

> *'I think that some people blame dairy and wheat intolerances because they don't eat very healthily the majority of the time, and these "intolerances" could be their excuses for a poorly balanced diet.'*
>
> **Catherine Hurley**

Our gastro-intestinal tracts, and the whole sequence of organs involved in digestion, are designed to receive a mixture of carbohydrates and proteins. When you start excluding foods, you cross into dangerous territory. Many vitamins are 'fat soluble', and if you eliminate fat, you interfere with the body's ability to absorb them.

High-protein diets cause the body to break down protein in a desperate attempt to create carbohydrates and, therefore, insulin. It's paradoxical that the person is eating protein but losing muscle.

Many people don't know the difference between allergies and intolerances. Forty per cent of Americans questioned in a recent survey felt they suffered from food allergies. The true figure is more likely to be 2 per cent! An allergy involves the immune system reacting swiftly to a substance, such as peanuts, which then causes it to produce a number of chemicals, such as histamine, to deal with the substance. Reactions are often dramatic and potentially fatal, ranging from swelling and breathing difficulties to extreme fatigue.

Intolerances, on the other hand, don't trigger the immune system and involve subtler reactions such as headaches, dark circles under eyes, poor concentration, bloated stomach, and aching muscles and joints.

Much of the hype and confusion about allergies and intolerances can be blamed on those seeking to profit from it, and some of the test kits you can buy are notoriously unreliable, with many people found to be sensitive to the foods they ate the day before. There is a strong case for tighter regulations of the industry, which is making huge profits from pseudo-science and then trying to sell follow-up supplements. One woman rang the chief executive of Allergy UK to say she had been told she was intolerant to 116 foods. She was living on rice pudding and had lost 19kg (42lb/3 stone) in a month.

TIP If you think you are intolerant to a specific type of food, cut down initially, rather than cutting it out completely. You may find you were simply overloading in that particular area.

If you feel strongly that wheat (or anything else) is a problem, choose an alternative in the same category, avoid the suspected source completely for one month (read food labels carefully while you do this), note the results, then reintroduce it, increasing the amount every day. If you notice any symptoms you should see your doctor. You may be one of the few who are genuinely intolerant to a certain food and need to be monitored professionally.

Eight signs of healthy eating

1. Eating three meals a day.
2. Occasionally overeating or undereating.
3. Using flexible restraint.
4. Eating a diverse, sufficient amount of food regularly to prevent bingeing.
5. Eating to 'watch your weight' rather than to always lose weight.
6. Knowing that eating well is important for good health.
7. Enjoying the experience of eating; finding it a pleasure.
8. Not using excuses of food intolerances to avoid eating well.

The winter blues

All supermodels know *that* feeling: tired, stressed – and craving carbohydrates. Those winter blues, caused partly by fluctuating hormone levels, affect hundreds of thousands of women, and the most common symptoms are overeating, particularly in the afternoon. A lot of us gain a few pounds in the colder months, usually during the Christmas holidays. The type of foods we eat also makes a major contribution to this weight gain. We're less likely to reach for a salad when we're chilly, and comfort foods are what we crave.

During the winter months outside activities lose their attraction, and our incentive to exercise drops off. We try to warm up our bodies by reaching for heavier foods and perhaps warming ourselves up with too much coffee. This becomes a vicious circle – it makes us jittery, and then we use food again to calm us down.

But why is 'the blues' syndrome so particular to women? Well, it's our old friend serotonin again. We have less effective receptors for this mood-enhancing brain chemical than men, and serotonin production is affected by oestrogen. When women have high oestrogen levels they have more serotonin activity, and when they have falling levels they have less. This is why women feel the body blues more acutely when they're premenstrual, after childbirth and during the menopause. Models know that the cure is staggeringly simple: getting plenty of bright light and taking moderate exercise can reverse many of the changes brought about by low or fluctuating hormones.

Bright light and moderate exercise boost serotonin activity, increase cerebral blood flow and reduce the level of stress hormones. As a result, you feel more energetic, think more clearly, have a better mood, eat less, feel more relaxed and cope with stress more effectively.

Light relief

We feel happier on sunny days because light enhances our mood, but most of us live a light-deprived existence. As soon as we leave home we duck into a car, bus or train. After work we rush home and spend most of our evenings cocooned indoors. But even a brightly lit room has only a fraction of the amount of light available outdoors during the day.

Our ancestors spent most of their time outdoors. They were woken by the sun, and the light stimulated the production of serotonin and other energising hormones. As a result their hearts beat faster, their metabolic rate increased and their minds became alert.

> *The sun makes me completely happy — I love it. My mother's Peruvian, so maybe that's why. I think it's important to let your skin breathe and not to get too uptight about it, and enjoy the elements.'*
>
> ### Helena Christensen

Getting more bright light each day by taking a morning walk, even in cloudy weather, has proved just as effective as sitting passively for two hours in front of a light box. Walking for just 20 minutes a day, five days a week can have an incredible effect. It lifts your spirits, which stops you reaching for food, increases your activity level, which helps you burn more calories, and suppresses your appetite, which lowers your calorie intake and boosts your metabolism.

TIP Light enters the body through the eyes. So if it's cloudy outside, or you're walking at the beginning or the end of the day, look for ways to increase your light exposure. Look at the brightest part of the sky from time to time, and look straight ahead rather than towards the ground.

Make the most of light levels indoors by opening all the blinds and curtains when you're at home. Cut back trees and shrubs that block the light, and arrange furniture so that you can sit close to a window and look outside. If you work at a desk for long periods make sure you face outside. Paint walls and ceilings light colours, and consider adding skylights and replacing small windows with larger ones. You can also increase artificial light by using fluorescent or high-wattage bulbs.

Exercising your head

Supermodels know they don't have to run, jog, lift weights, sweat, join a gym, buy special equipment, wear a skimpy leotard or even change clothes to enhance their mood through exercise. All they need to do is just whack on a comfortable pair of shoes, open the door and start walking. Halfway through their first walk they begin to enjoy the 'walker's high'. Regular brisk walking is just as good a way to enhance your mood as more intense exercise, such as jogging or running, but without the sweat. Walk for ten minutes in one direction, then turn round and come back. Within just a few minutes of brisk walking your heart begins to beat more rapidly and, as your heart rate increases, more blood flows to your brain. This increased blood flow enhances your ability to think and concentrate, and within 10 to 15 minutes into your walk, blood circulation in your brain has increased by up to 50 per cent. After 20 minutes your mental fog begins to lift and your mood moves up several notches. For the next few hours, you'll feel less anxious, happier and more energetic.

Many women turn to food to experience these same good feelings, but walking is a far better way to generate a sustained sense of well-being. A study that compared the effects of eating a sweet snack with going for a brisk ten-minute walk found the sugar high lasted for only about 30 minutes, after which the women felt more tired and tense than they had before eating it. But when the same people went for a brisk walk, they felt better for several hours afterwards, without experiencing a dip in mood or energy levels. When you walk briskly for just 20 minutes a day, five days a week, you could lose as much as 11 pounds a year – without dieting. You will also be losing fat, not muscle.

> *'It's scientifically recognised that how you think and feel is influenced by the levels of vitality you experience. Your endorphins react to sunlight – walking in the fresh air is very good for the brain cells.'*
>
> **Catherine Hurley**

Walking also gives you an amazing, glowing appearance, tones your muscles and improves your posture. Remember to think 'tall' as you walk. Imagine there's a string attached to the top of your head that is pulling you up and elongating your spine. Pull up your ribcage so that you increase the distance between the bottom of your ribs and your waist. After just six to eight weeks of regular walking and getting more light, you'll find this has proved a reliable way of producing mood-enhancing chemicals, which will override your need for food to boost your energy levels. You'll be relieving your symptoms through your own effort and determination, and you'll be able to use walking whenever you need to release stress. You'll be lighter in mood, lighter on your feet, less tense and super-positive.

Sunshine machines

Used by some models who spend endless hours under studio lights rather than daylight, the light box is a useful invention if your job often stops you from seeing the light (so it could be more useful than you think!). It's also used by many of the women who suffer from Seasonal Affective Disorder (SAD), and it involves sitting close to a special light box for between 30 minutes and two hours a day.

You need to be exposed to a minimum dose of around 2,500 lux (a measurement of brightness). Ordinary domestic or office lighting emits only about 200–500 lux. On a bright summer's day the intensity can be up to 100,000 lux.

Some light boxes double as an alarm clock by waking you with a sunrise imitation, others can be carried around like a briefcase or worn like a sun visor so you can use it while you're doing other things, such as having breakfast. Light boxes are useful as an alternative to sunlight if you're house- or office-bound, and some companies offer them on a trial basis, or you can hire or buy them. A word of warning, however: many of these machines don't reach the minimum lux requirement, so check that they at least reach 2,500 and preferably 5,000–10,000 lux.

'I will' power

It's easy to think that Kate Moss, Claudia Schiffer, and all the other model mums who bounce back with incredible, streamlined figures within weeks of giving birth have some magical secret combined with incredible willpower. The truth is they manage to regain their figures quickly because they know it's easier to do something straight away than to let it run away with them. The process of achieving goals occurs the second you start making them real.

> **TIP** Be confident. Confident people think they can succeed, and they do. If you think you can't you won't.

Supermodels know they have to get back to work. Having a good body is what they do for a living; they are their own product – and they want it enough to make sure they do it. The only difference between supermodels and other women is that models make a living from the way they look, so they try that bit harder. If you don't believe me, think of a time when you aimed for something great and succeeded: passed your driving test, scored a job you wanted or a man you fancied. Consider how you did it, because the technique works for anything. Ask yourself:

- What motivated you to achieve this goal?

- How did you keep going when you wanted to give up?

- What or who did you get to help you, and why?

Willpower isn't really something you have or don't have; it's a skill. It's a sign that you've made a conscious choice to do something based on your thoughts about the consequences of that choice or action.

Motivation is an important part of a top model's life. She'll make sure she eats and exercises in a way she knows will promote the right production of hormones and brain chemicals to keep motivated. Remember: when your brain is motivated, healthy food actually tastes great, and you want to eat it. And when healthy food is more satisfying, it's no longer an effort to choose it over junk food.

'It's not about looking good; it's about being 100 per cent honest to yourself about being healthy. That means eating organic food whenever possible and making an effort not to eat processed food, to drink water and not drink alcohol. It's easy to kid yourself, but what's the point in that?'
Elle Macpherson

Find someone who has achieved what you want to achieve – it's essential to stay inspired. Connect with other people who are also conscious about their health.

Be aware of the benefits you'll personally reap when you achieve your aim.

Think what would happen if you didn't – how bad you'd be feeling a year from now.

4

Why quick-fix diets don't work for models

Every season hundreds of new diet books are published: in summer it's how to look great in a bikini, pre-Christmas it's drop three sizes to fit into your festive frock and then, surprise, surprise, it's New Year's resolution time. The same old diets, the same tired advice disguised and re-hashed to appear exciting and new. The problem with these books is that they always give you a short-term goal to focus on. Having reached your target and with no sustaining strategies, you regain the weight you lost. All your hard work undone. Dieting with a short-term goal only ever gives you short-term results. It's a total con.

A top model's livelihood depends on remaining a consistent dress size for the entire duration of her career while she constantly travels the international circuit of Paris, London, Milan and New York. It's not an option for her to concoct special meals with great care, always count calories, obsess about combining some foods and not others, constantly leap on the scales or have imagined wheat/dairy intolerances. Most diet books and programmes are so complicated and difficult to follow that the majority of dieters become literally consumed with thoughts of food and how to figure out what to eat next. It's only when they finally sit down to a meal that naturally appeals to them that they feel like a real person again. Supermodels don't have the time or inclination to eat abnormally and obsessively, which a restrictive diet demands. Whether they eat on planes, in studios, on location, in hotels, restaurants or at home, it's a given that they simply search out the healthiest food available to help maintain their stamina and keep their looks intact.

There's nothing precious about these girls – they drink a bit, sometimes smoke a bit and occasionally eat comfort food. It's laughable to believe they 'only eat rabbit food' – or worse. This is a convenient myth perpetuated by sensation seekers and jealous wannabes. Does Kate Moss look as though she deprives herself? Come and see the vast quantities of healthy food I sell to well-known models at my deli!

Obviously exceptions do exist, but no reputable model agency will keep a girl on their books – however beautiful– if she exhibits emotional baggage with drugs or food. They simply don't need the hassle. There are hundreds of lovely, professional, reliable girls out there from whom they can take their commission.

'I always tell new young models that they won't work in the marketplace if they get too thin.

Magazines and advertising clients simply won't want to use them.'

Sarah Doukas
Storm Model Agent

In ten years of modelling in Paris, Milan, London and New York, I never came across a top girl who was a problem eater. None of the models interviewed for this book have special diets or food idiosyncrasies. True, busy models sometimes don't eat as regularly as they should because they're working hard, but it's the same for secretaries.

'It's simply not true that girls are pushed to be skinny. I follow a healthy-eating regime, but once I was laid up with flu and lost a stone. My agency were horrified when they saw me, and told me not to come back until I'd put it back on.'

Jacqui Ainsley
Bond girl

Forget the fads

If you want to lose weight, the last thing you need is a one-dimensional diet book telling you what to do. It works best when you make your own choices on how to survive the seductive minefield of excess food.

TIP Eat nurturing food to make your body work more efficiently. Then let your body – not some stupid chart – tell you what your weight should be. The right weight for you will make you feel healthy, energetic, and confident, and it will be easy to maintain. The chances are if you've never been a size eight, you're not meant to be!

Okay, it's true some people have these skills naturally, but others get this 'control' by working it out themselves, rather than following rigid plans. Successful slimmers are nearly always the ones who take useful and sensible information from a variety of sources and use it to develop their own healthy weight-loss strategies. A recent American survey revealed that 72 per cent of women who had lost weight (on average 15kg (33lb/2 stone 5 lb)), and kept it off, had ultimately done it on their own, compared to only 20 per cent in commercial slimming groups. Those who maintained their lost weight used the classic weight-loss strategies: being more active, eating more healthily and having smaller portions, and they found ways of fitting these skills into their lives, rather than following rigid diets. To keep on track, the women set themselves small targets they could meet and stuck to plans they made personally from various sources until their new habits were established. They ate regular meals, had very few snacks, and eventually discovered they didn't want to eat as much, and that very fatty and sweet foods lost their regular appeal. They also switched to low-fat cooking methods, ate more fruit and vegetables, confronted their problems directly rather than avoiding them and acknowledged support from friends, family or health professionals (not slimming clubs!).

How not to lose weight

- *Follow rigid diets you can't sustain.*
- *Eat snacks, especially confectionery.*
- *Use formula diets, appetite suppressants, or fast.*
- *Never or rarely exercise.*
- *Skip breakfast.*
- *Ban favourite (high-fat) foods and feel deprived.*
- *View diet foods differently from what you really want to eat.*
- *Eat differently from your family.*
- *Eat in response to a negative life event.*
- *Eat in a subconscious response to emotions.*
- *Never or rarely confront problems directly.*
- *Never or rarely use the support of others.*

Set point

The weight at which your body tends to hover naturally is medically called your 'set point' – something like a thermostat in a central-heating system. It's often blamed for the inability to lose weight. When we pig out, our metabolism speeds up to burn off the excess food. But when we reduce our intake, such as when we go on a diet, our body goes into survival mode, slowing down our metabolism. If we continually diet, our body thermostat eventually fails to reset itself once we begin eating normally again. Our metabolism continues to operate at the slow rate and we start to regain weight. This leads to the 'yo-yo' effect – a vicious cycle of weight gain and weight loss.

To lower your 'set point', it's best to maintain any weight loss for at least a year. Until then your body will do all it can to get your weight back up to its heavier set point, which is why we crave food and then binge. It takes time to change your habits and convince your body that it's a change for life.

Never say diet

What can I say about the high-profile, high-protein diets where you fill yourself with saturated fats for extended periods of time, that hasn't been said before? We all know they work in the short term, if you can stand it, but the down side is pretty unpleasant and the long-term effects are unknown.

The slow-moving transit of animal fat through the gut, and lack of fibre, is uncomfortable at best and may increase the risk of bowel cancer and heart disease. The low levels of carbohydrate in these diets can reduce the levels of serotonin, one of the chemicals that regulates mood and encourages relaxed and positive feelings. The problem is magnified in women because they have naturally lower levels of serotonin, so this diet can lead to irritability and even depression, as well as possible physical complications.

'Restrictive diets are incredibly dangerous for young girls to be involved with. I certainly would never recommend any of the models on my books try them — they're far too extreme and unnecessary. A healthy diet and regular exercise is so simple and natural to incorporate into your life.'

Sarah Doukas
Storm Model Agent

But the most important aspect of these high-protein, restrictive diets is that they can suit some people and not others – there is no in-between – and no knowing if your body will react violently against it until you do it. Deviating from the Atkins diet in any way during the first two weeks can be dangerous and can seriously damage your body. The vice-president of the Atkins Health Service, Collette Heimowitz, has stated that 'when you cheat with alcohol, or bread etc., you are switching back to a carbohydrate metabolism, which is a different metabolism, so high carb, high fat is the most deadliest of combinations'. It seems to me that this diet is best suited to the carbohydrate-sensitive people who've had a tendency to be overweight for most of their lives, and who get less hungry by eating large amounts of protein.

On the other hand, a calorie-sensitive person who is overweight by less than 11.3kg (25lb/1 stone 11lb) and doesn't have the symptoms associated with poor carbohydrate metabolism – food cravings which disappear when they eat starchy or sugary foods – will not be successful with this diet, and may even gain a few pounds.

> *'I went on the Atkins diet. It was horrendous. I was only doing it to help my PA. We both said okay – no more chocolate, but I love chocolate. We lasted three days!'*
>
> **Jodie Kidd**

The fried breakfast heaven of one group is the retching nightmare of another. But the phenomenal success of high-protein diets is surely based on the concept that they're diets that don't seem like diets, because you can eat lots of greasy, stodgy things. You can have the forbidden fruit. Well, not actual fruit, obviously, but mountains of meat covered in cream and butter. A major concern when cutting out fruit and many vegetables from your diet is getting enough vitamins and minerals, but these diets advise taking supplements instead. In fact the sale of the books is matched by the sale of the nutritional supplements manufactured to take with the eating programme. Inevitably, food manufacturers everywhere are getting in on the act. In America there are now 800 special foods available labelled 'low carb' – ketchup, cereal bars, milkshakes, chocolate, bread, and so on. The problem is that there is no definition of what exactly can, and what can't, be labelled low carbohydrate. The Foods Standards Agency has issued guidelines about what can be called low fat, reduced fat and virtually fat-free. However, no such guidelines exist for the carbohydrate content of foods.

> **TIP** An Atkins Advantage chocolate bar costs far more than a standard bar, and yet contains roughly the same fat and calories, so it won't help you lose weight unless you follow a very strict low-carb regime.

There's also the chance that people who aren't overweight will think that these kinds of foods are a healthier alternative to normal food. They're not. They won't reduce your waistline but they'll always reduce your bank balance. Still, if you're the kind of person prepared to take a potentially dangerous risk to get slim, rather than choosing a less violent way of losing weight, and always have cauliflowers in your cupboard instead of potatoes, prefer tofu to bananas, enjoy fried eggs for breakfast, steak for lunch and cheesy snacks, then you too can be a contender. And I won't make any unfair, ungracious and biased comments about your breath smelling like a sumo wrestler's jock strap, because you may be one of the very few whose doesn't.

Hard-to-swallow diet options

All diets promote one type of food to be eaten while outlawing others. But then there are the food-combining diets, whose main principle is that you should never eat carbohydrates (pasta, bread, rice, potatoes, and so on) in the same meal as proteins (meat, fish, some dairy products, beans, and so on). The belief here is that the digestive system tends to lay down fat more easily when protein and carbs are eaten together. If you keep them in separate meals your weight will find its natural balance. Four hours should be left between consuming any starch and protein foods – but egg yolks, nuts, cream, and seeds can be eaten with starch or protein. Well, that's all right then. Not complicated or impractical at all. But I think I can resist. For some reason I always enjoy meat and potatoes, or curry and rice on the same plate at the same time. I'm funny that way.

> **TIP** Don't ever consider buying diet pills from shops, ads or the Internet. Many of them contain ephedrine: a powerful nervous system stimulant that carries a host of side effects, ranging from tremors and insomnia to heart attacks and strokes. The pills that don't contain ephedrine don't make enough of a difference to be worth their expensive outlay.

Weight Watchers sell you the idea that life will become a whole lot better if you join them. Many people do. You pay an initial registration fee and a weekly fee to attend a weigh-in and meeting of up to an hour, and its programme is based on a points system. Food and drinks are given a value, based on their saturated fat and calorie content, and members are then allocated a maximum number of daily points, depending on their weight, with the aim of reaching a specific target. But if it worked, surely their customers would only have to sign up once. Instead it relies on clients returning to its diet programmes and products over and over again. The few who do lose weight permanently can be claimed as victory and photographed for publicity. The Duchess of York is their biggest success story, but then she has the ultimate powerful incentive to stay in shape – a £1 million-a-year contract with Weight Watchers in the US. Wouldn't we all do it if we were being paid a million quid?

Three generations of supermodels who have never dieted

··

> *'I've never thought that dieting works, though changing the way you eat has enormous benefits.'*
>
> ### Catherine Hurley

> *'I don't diet because it destroys your metabolism. I eat three meals a day and I try not to eat in between. All the food I eat is organic.'*
>
> ### Claudia Schiffer

> *'I eat three balanced meals every day — if you skip meals, your body just stores fat. I don't snack and do my best to avoid too much alcohol.'*
>
> ### Jerry Hall

Then there are the meal-substitute diets where you replace two meals a day with the company's packaged, dried products – milkshakes, soups, pasta, and so on. I haven't had the pleasure of tasting any of these powdered delicacies but you must drink two shakes a day for six months and the cereal bars are covered in chocolate (not exactly the right message) for which you pay several hundred smackers. Pass.

The South Beach Diet is high-protein, but distinguishes between healthy fats and artery-clogging ones. It puts a ban on high glycaemic index (GI) food, which makes blood-sugar levels rise quickly, then fall (so that you crave more carbs again) and it's concept is spreading as a popular theme for many current diet books – all following similar ideas with a focus on blood-sugar spikes and crashes. Their authors claim that if you eat low GI foods your body actually stores less fat, but, according to a professor of nutrition interviewed for this book, there is no scientific evidence to prove this. Nor is there any proof that eating low GI foods necessarily leads to weight loss. You might eat a baked potato with cheese or a salad and this combination will actually alter its GI. Even the temperature at which you eat food matters – a hot mashed potato has a higher GI than a colder one!

'I try to eat organic foods as much as possible, but basically my philosophy is to try and eat food that makes me strong and happy. I believe a healthy body will let you know what food it needs.'

Elle Macpherson

These diets assume that a steady blood-sugar level stops you overeating, but cravings are only one reason why we eat too much. Not a word is given about the psychological reasons. Still, they're healthier than some diets – at least they encourage whole grains and a mix of protein, fruit and vegetables.

Followers of the Raw-food Diet, popular with the Hollywood fraternity, claim that heating food above about 46ºC (116ºF) destroys healthy enzymes and they, therefore, eat about 75 per cent of their food uncooked. But when you cook a carrot you increase the amount of the enzyme beta-carotene, a form of vitamin A that helps your eyes and immune system; cooked tomatoes contain more antioxidants than uncooked ones, so can protect you against certain types of cancer. Essentially, however, this diet seems more attractive than most, but who really wants a carrot stick for lunch in the dead of winter?

'I don't believe in diets — I instinctively know what's good for me, and that a little bit of what isn't doesn't hurt. I am naturally hyperactive so I need protein and fats for energy. I get run down if I don't eat properly, so I never skip meals.'

Laura Bailey

What unites all the crazy diets is that their effectiveness is only temporary. It's almost impossible to live a punishing guilt-ridden life of self-denial, and virtually everyone gives up. But this doesn't stop people believing there's a quick fix out there somewhere that will allow them to eat until they're stuffed, do the minimum exercise and still lose weight. But there isn't.

'When you cut things out, that's when you crave them. Moderation and balance is the only way that makes sense. If you're happy about the way you live your life then true beauty shows through. It's got nothing to do with your eating habits.'

India Hicks

Why eating well is the best revenge

The major food industries and diet promoters have a vested interest in hyping up our focus on food: the first by piling on the pounds with their highly addictive, chemically enhanced products and the latter by telling us how to remove them. It suits the diet industry to convince us that we need their goods. They think they have a captive market psychologically prepared for them by the media, fashion and advertising industries, which constantly bombard us with photographs of slim women. It's time we returned to a much healthier relationship with food and body image. The relentless pursuit of skinniness has brought only misery and guilt. Fad dieting, whether fat-free, carb-free or liquid filled, makes your face look gaunt and lacklustre faster than smoking, sun exposure and stress.

Psychologists have found that women on diets show poorer memory, slower reaction times, inability to maintain attention and poorer planning ability than those who aren't, and that trying to lose weight can bring on a range of symptoms associated with clinical depression and anxiety. But gradually the tide is turning. Women are not the stupid creatures the diet industry thinks they are. For most women, the chief preoccupation in life is not the pursuit of a size eight frock. It's the Nigella Lawsons of this world, with their laid-back, confident attitude to their looks, and a love of good food, who are fast becoming the new icons for many women – and certainly for men.

Women are craving honesty in their busy, productive lives. Constantly bombarded with beauty products, alternative therapies, spas, designer clothes and all manner of gizmos to persuade them to look more beautiful, they do not want to be disillusioned or waste time on nutri-babble that tries to sell them a dream that doesn't work. On the other hand, women want fantasy too. That is why glossy, sophisticated magazines exist. They represent a few minutes of escapism where nothing is real, including the models. We want to see the models airbrushed to perfection, wearing ridiculously expensive clothes. We love seeing accessories photographed like precious museum pieces. When magazines toyed with using older, more 'real' model girls, surveys told them that women didn't want that – they want to dream about perfection.

'I could keep on modelling till I'm 85 with the digital adjustments I know how to do. After every shoot I pull the photographer aside and say, "You will be retouching, right?" If they say, "Only if there's a budget," I immediately suggest they scan the pictures for me to retouch. People

see the images and think you're a goddess, when the reality is different.'

Lisa B

Many supermodels are not beautiful in real life; they simply photograph beautifully. There are very few you would recognise when they are off-duty. Those chic, young women gliding down Bond Street and Park Avenue dressed head-to-toe in designer labels are never models, but the trophy wives of rich men, or fashionista women who make their living from fashion, such as stylists and magazine writers. Supermodels wear jeans, T-shirts and comfortable anonymous jackets!

'You'll never be pretty but you'll always be magnificent.'

Angelica Houston to Erin O'Connor

The tide is turning. Women are wising up, acquiring a more intelligent and less emotional approach to 'physical perfection' and learning the vital difference between self-maintenance and self-obsession. They know they need to be slim, not thin, or their bodies will fight them all the way. Women are more aware than ever before that there are enormously powerful 'feelgood' industries out there (and many small alternative ones) tapping into their 'body image' insecurities and laughing all the way to the bank.

Part Two
The Fresh Way

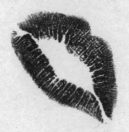

'Discovering good food is like discovering good
sex: once you get the taste for it there's no going
back.'

India Hicks
Supermodel and marathon runner
Campaigns: Ralph Lauren Fragrance, Gap,
Bill Blass, Banana Republic

5

How to recognise good food

'You are what you eat,' said Yoko Ono, and I remember that existential moment when I realised what she meant: that food you swallowed didn't simply disappear down your throat, but stayed decomposing in your gut for up to 72 hours. At some point it dawns on you – where does the food go? It didn't exactly stop me wanting to eat everything that took my fancy, although I refrained from having intimate relationships with hot dogs and frankfurters. There was not, however, a biblical conversion to the offerings of health-food stores.

What is it about those places? They all have the same distinctive smell, a cross between countless dried pulses and embalming fluid – their offerings, worthy things to be endured rather than enjoyed, and sadly lacking in the 'eat me now' factor. Most models would rather chew their own arms than live on tofu stir-fry, cottage cheese and mung beans, ridiculously healthy though they are. There's an enormous difference between good food that tastes sexy and luscious, and food that 'does you good' but tastes like rush matting. Take fruit for example: we should be eating at least two portions every day, but it's not easy when fruit rarely tastes as inviting as it looks. That shiny supermarket apple, so perfect it could have been painted by Cézanne, tastes … well, it tastes of the wax that makes it shine.

For the large food retailers, the supermarkets, it's the visual impact that counts. In their eyes we buy with our eyes. We used to get local seasonal produce from market traders and greengrocers, but, thanks to supermarkets, seasons don't exist any more for fresh fruit and vegetables. Today, retailers can source food from wherever it's cheapest around the globe at the touch of a computer key. You can have anything you want, at any time – it comes into the country as refrigerated cargo and is ripened in transit. But, despite its appearance of near perfection, there is a huge price to pay. The further afield fruit travels and the longer the time spent at low temperatures, the more the vitamin and mineral contents deteriorate, and the end result is likely to be slushy and flavourless.

The good news is that many of the best fruit growers sell their produce themselves through local markets, friendly greengrocers and farmers' markets. Or you can be really pro-active and visit local pick-your-own farms, where you can pluck your own organic produce rather than purchasing tasteless, air-freighted rubbish. But what do you do if you only have a supermarket or corner shop handy? You learn how to choose fruit that will give you the ripest maximum return imaginable. If that sounds as though you're doing some long-term investing in a precious commodity, well you are.

Sexing up your fruit

There's nothing more sensuous than a downy, blushing peach with its bulging, round, fleshy cheeks, exquisite smell and juice running down your chin when you bite into it, and that incredible ... sorry, where was I?

Sniffing your chosen fruit is one of the best ways to tell how ripe a fruit was when it was picked: the more fragrant it smells, the riper it is. Most harvested fruits don't ripen nearly as well as they would on the tree, vine or bush, and some don't ripen at all! Strangely, most vegetables have weak, uncomplicated aromas until you cook them.

> **TIP** Eat fruit instead of sugar. Think of a mouth-watering piece of fruit as your sugar. Take the ripest, therefore the sweetest, piece of fruit and eat it at room temperature, for maximum flavour and satisfaction.

Peaches, apples and bananas *ripen after they are picked*. Mature peaches, nectarines, plums and apricots shouldn't have any traces of green. Also, ignore the red blush new varieties, which have been bred to turn red long before they're ripe. Some of the sweetest juiciest peaches and nectarines never colour beyond bright yellow.

Fruits that *never ripen after they are picked* are black-berries, cherries, dates, grapes, grapefruit, lemons, mandarins, oranges, pineapples, raspberries, strawberries and watermelons. Buy them ripe, store them with care and wash them only before serving to avoid damaging their skins and inviting decay.

Fruits that *ripen in colour, texture and juiciness but don't improve in sweetness or flavour after they are picked* are apricots, blueberries, cantaloupes, figs, honeydews, nectarines, passion fruit, peaches and plums.

Fruits that do *get sweeter after harvest* are apples, kiwis, mangoes, papayas and pears. Apples and pears sweeten up very well. In fact, pears become mushy when ripened completely on the tree.

Bananas are *picked when mature but completely green*, so buy them green if you've time to let them ripen. Hard green bananas are less likely to have been injured in handling than those softened and yellowed along the way. Buy them with the stems fully attached and without splits in the skin. Ripen them in a paper bag until completely yellow.

> **TIP** Hold a grape in your mouth before chewing it very, very slowly. Taste how deliciously refreshing it becomes as it explodes in your mouth. Now hold a crisp in your mouth and feel the overwhelming oil slick it's created.

Melons are the nectar of the gods and, together with berries, are the favourite fruit of supermodels – especially the cantaloupe and honeydew. One half of a cantaloupe melon provides more vitamin A (beta-carotene) and vitamin C than most other fruits. It's also high in potassium, has wonderful orange flesh and is only 95 calories per serving.

You must choose a melon wisely in order to experience its perfect, clean taste. Choose a cantaloupe with a thick, close netting and avoid those with smooth areas or soft mushy spots. When it's ripe and ready, the stem scar will be smooth and the ends will yield slightly to the pressure of your finger. If the stem is still attached or the scar is jagged, it was taken from the vine too early. If it's too hard it will never ripen properly or become sweet enough.

Watermelon champagne — every supermodel's favourite

Don't drive after eating!

Take one large, washed watermelon and a bottle of champagne (pink, if you like) or a good dry sparkling white or rosé wine. Cut a small hole in the top of the melon and scoop out 2 tablespoons of flesh. Then pour in as much champagne as you can. Leave to marinate for a day and then add more champagne to saturate it again.

To serve: cut the melon into small chunks and serve mixed with raspberries, blueberries or black grapes.

Honeydew melons are slightly larger, and have a yellowish-white smooth skin with a light green flesh inside. Test for ripeness in the same way as cantaloupes. If you can't find one ripe enough, allow it to stand at room temperature until ripe, then store it in the fridge.

It's important to scrub the rind of all melons with a mild detergent, as they can carry bacteria and mould, and thoroughly rinse before cutting into the flesh.

Very juicy citrus fruits are firm and heavy for their size. The colour of oranges isn't important, but look for the small, flower-shaped button at one end: if it's green, the orange was picked recently, or handled well, or both. A dark, brittle button indicates good-bye, rather than good buy.

Catherine Hurley's fresh raspberry fool

Wash 250g (9oz) fresh raspberries thoroughly and then stew with a little clear honey until the juice from the fruit has just started to run. Remove from the heat and allow to cool. Mix the raspberries very gently with plain yoghurt and leave to chill. Divide among four tall glasses and serve.

If the hard-skinned fruit you buy is organic, simply wash it in warm running water using a soft vegetable brush before eating. If it's not organic, wash more thoroughly to get rid of chemical residues, and soak in cold water for ten minutes. You can eat the skin of most fruits – it contains valuable nutrients, but don't eat the skin of a heavily waxed apple. Wax doesn't dissolve when cleaned with water.

Remove the rinds of citrus fruit, but eat the white part inside the skin for its vitamin C and bioflavonoid content.

Fruity tips

Increase your enjoyment of fruit with these taste-improving ideas:

- Enhance the flavour of strawberries by splashing on a little balsamic vinegar or sprinkling with finely ground black pepper.

- Speed up the ripening of soft fruits, such as peaches, by storing them overnight in a box covered in newspaper, or in a paper bag with a ripe banana or apple.

- Don't remove the stalks and leaves from strawberries until after they have been washed or they will become mushy.

- Keep sliced or chopped apples and pears from turning brown by dipping them into a bowl of acidulated water (water with a few drops of lemon or vinegar in it).

- If you're serving melon or papaya as part of an appetiser, add a tiny amount of lime juice and a little salt and pepper to bring out the sweet, juicy flavour.

- Always buy unwaxed or organic lemons when you want to use the zest or rind.

- One lemon yields about 3 tablespoons of juice and about 2 teaspoons of grated zest.

- Submerge lemons in hot water 15 minutes before squeezing, to yield almost twice the amount of juice.

- If you use only half a lemon, freeze the rest – just pop it into a freezer bag and save to use later.

- Soak dried fruit in boiling water for a few minutes to soften it and kill any bacteria or mould that forms during the drying process.

What makes food 'organic'?

When it hasn't had chemical fertilisers, insecticides, fungicides, herbicides or pesticides sprayed on it, or any post-harvest treatment, such as waxing, food can be classed as organic. In the case of meat, the animals must not be given medicine such as antibiotics, and they must feed on pesticide-free food. It's an offence to use the word 'organic' unless the produce has been certified by a recognised organic agency.

Chart your fruit benefits

FRUIT	BENEFIT
Apple	reactivates beneficial gut bacteria, reduces cholesterol
Apricot	potent antioxidant, natural sweetener and laxative
Banana	promotes sleep, mild laxative, anti-fungal, natural antibiotic
Blackberry	tonic and blood cleanser, relieves diarrhoea
Blueberry	laxative, blood cleanser, improves circulation, benefits eyesight
Cherry	anti-spasmodic, relieves headaches, natural antiseptic

Cranberry	kills bacteria and viruses in kidneys, bladder and urinary tract
Date	protects against diarrhoea, dysentery and respiratory problems
Fig	laxative, restorative, increases vitality, clears toxins, high in calcium
Grapefruit	blood cleanser, fights allergies and infections of the throat and mouth
Kiwi	removes excess sodium from the body, excellent source of vitamin C
Lemon/Lime	astringent, potent antiseptic, great for colds, coughs, sore throats
Mango	blood cleanser, combats acidity and poor digestion. Good for kidneys
Melon	great cleanser and rehydrator. Eat on its own for maximum benefits
Orange	excellent antiseptic, cleanses from within
Papaya	aids digestion, anti-cancer, soothes intestinal gas, detoxifier
Peach	cleanses kidneys and bladder, laxative, diuretic
Pear	high iodine content, diuretic, helps remove toxins
Pineapple	has potent digestive enzyme that consumes bacteria and parasites
Prune	laxative, good for blood, brain and nerves. Helps lower cholesterol
Raspberry	relieves menstrual cramps, helps expel mucus, phlegm, toxins
Strawberry	anti-cancer, antiviral, antibacterial

Avocados — the perfect food

Most people think of avocados as vegetables. This may account for the astonishing fact that two-thirds of people in this country have never ever tasted an avocado. It's the most nutritious of all fruit eaten raw and is known as 'the perfect food' because it's high in unsaturated (good) fat, full of minerals, not especially calorific and contains all the antioxidant vitamins. Easily digested, it aids blood and tissue regeneration and is rarely sprayed by growers. Perfect!

These days avocados are very affordable, but back in the 1950s, when they were considered highly exotic, they retailed at Harrods for £10 each. I prefer the pebble-textured, almost black, Hass variety, which has fewer fibres and is much more buttery than the green Fuerte. During the UK summer, look for the South African avocados, with wonderful, creamy flesh. An avocado travels well and ripens only after it has been picked. You must ripen it at room temperature, and it will keep for up to ten days in the fridge. The ripening process can be speeded up by placing a banana next to your avocado. If you buy an unripened avocado and you need it in a hurry, put it in a microwave oven on medium for about 45 seconds, rotating halfway. You won't ripen it, but it will be softer.

The easy way to enjoy an avocado

Cut the fruit in half lengthways. Take out the stone and pour in some Worcestershire sauce. Add a twist of black pepper and eat slowly with a spoon.

Fruity ... moi?

Strictly speaking, tomatoes are also fruits, but in practice they're the most popular vegetable we use – and the most abused! The poor, old, ubiquitous tomato is sold all year round and we tend to chuck them in the fridge until we need them. But that's exactly where they shouldn't go. It keeps them underripe and tasteless. Refrigeration kills any sweet, natural fruitiness, especially in summer, when they may actually have ripened in the sun. Who wants to eat them rock hard and stone cold? You can, however, freeze tomatoes whole for cooking. The skins will slip off easily when they have defrosted.

Originally cultivated in South America, Mexico and the Galapagos Islands more than 1,200 years ago, when they grew in yellow, green, white and black, as well as red, tomatoes are one of the richest sources of vitamin A – essential for the production of female sex hormones and for promoting fertility. They're also a good source of vitamin C and are rich in lycopene, a flavonoid that appears to reduce the risk of many cancers. Tomatoes also aid in the cleansing of toxins and protect against digestive disorders. Fresh, vine-ripened ones are best.

Know your tomatoes

CHERRY AND COCKTAIL Tiny tomatoes, round or plum-shaped, available in red, orange and yellow with an intense sweet flavour. Usually eaten raw in salads but can be briefly cooked and blended to make a quick sauce. Wonderful grilled or roasted. Try injecting them with a syringe full of vodka mixed with some Worcestershire sauce and Tabasco for a little Bloody Mary cocktail treat.

PLUM The most common variety is the Roma. It's a favourite with chefs because its skin is tough, which makes it easy to peel and then dice for cooking.

BEEFSTEAK Large and round, with fewer seeds and meatier flesh. Beefsteak tomatoes have less flavour than other varieties unless they're from Sicily, Italy or Cyprus.

ROUND These are sold on the vine and are even claimed to be 'grown for flavour'. They don't necessarily taste any better, however.

GREEN Either picked green and used for chutneys, or specially grown, generally in Italy, and suitable for salsas and salads.

GOLDEN, YELLOW AND ORANGE Come in all shapes and sizes and also in tiny cherry form. Treat them like red tomatoes.

TOMATILLO South American tomatoes, which look more like cape gooseberries with a protective skin that is removed before eating. They're quite sweet and don't have many seeds, making them perfect for salsas.

TAMARILLO Generally used as a fruit. It's oval and has a thick deep-red skin. Inside it's deep orange with black seeds. The flesh is very tart and requires cooking.

A sauce to source

In summer when tomatoes are abundant, and the heat means they won't keep for long, make a trip to your local market or greengrocer and haggle for loads of squishy tomatoes, which would otherwise be thrown out. They'll make the most fantastic, top-value tomato sauce you've ever tasted.

METHOD

1 Simply soften one chopped onion and one garlic clove in 15ml (1 tbsp) olive oil for every 450g (1lb) of tomatoes. Add some basil, salt, pepper and then the roughly chopped tomatoes. Don't worry about the seeds and skins, but do remove the woody part at the top.

2 Simmer for about 2 hours and then allow to cool. Blitz the mixture in a blender, sieve to remove the seeds, and freeze. The flavour is unbeatable – your boring old pasta tubes with tomato sauce will magically morph into *penne al pomodoro* and you'll have the taste of Tuscany all year round.

The cruciferous belters that know they're not fruits

The Magnificent Twelve cruciferous vegetables, so called because they all have flowers with four petals, which botanical historians describe as resembling the crucifix, have incredible powers to fight cancer and heart disease – the top two killers in the Western world. These vegetables are the most important of all the foods on our planet. Packed with vitamins, minerals, enzymes, fibre, protein and all the nutrients you need for a healthy body, they've been eaten by nearly every culture since time began. Okay, I've got wind of the fact that gobbling on a Brussels sprout is not as sensuous as canoodling with a peach, but sometimes it's cosy to be hearty not haute; let's face it, there are times in our lives when comforting scrambled eggs on toast hits the mark a lot more effectively than edgy seared tuna on rocket.

The Magnificent Twelve

VEGETABLE	BENEFITS
Broccoli	calcium, magnesium, phosphorus, high in vitamin C, folic acid
Brussels sprouts	rich in vitamins A, C, riboflavin, iron, potassium, fibre
Cabbage	excellent blood purifier, kills bacteria and viruses
Cauliflower	rich in vitamin C, potassium and fibre, blood purifier
Horseradish	digestive stimulant, aids lymphatic congestion
Kale	best cancer-fighting vegetable on the planet, protects against osteoporosis
Kohlrabi	high amounts of calcium, vitamin C, potassium, fibre

Mustard greens	crammed with iron, calcium, vitamin A
Radish	stimulates appetite, good for colds and flu, cleanses liver and gall bladder
Swede (rutabaga)	deep roots draw many nutrients from the earth, good for congestion, contains anti-cancer properties
Turnip	high in calcium, iron, niacin, good eaten raw or in salads. Steam the tops
Watercress	high in vitamin A, iron, calcium, copper, magnesium, iodine

Green piece

All supermodels know the importance of incorporating a diverse selection of vegetables into their diet. Whether eaten raw, steamed, boiled, baked, or sautéed, vegetables give us a broad spectrum of tastes and textures – sweet, salty, bitter, soft, chewy and crunchy.

Cook with more stems and leaves, mix your colours to get a variety of nutrients – and remember the darker the green, the more intense the nutrient content. Vegetables add fibre and flavour to your life; they're extraordinary immune boosters, slowing down the ageing process and preventing disease, but the best thing of all is that they have a remarkably low calorie and fat count, so you can eat all you like, whenever you like.

TIP Become aware of your relationship with food. Sit down and take notice of your food with all your senses – how it looks, smells, feels and tastes in your mouth. If you make time to eat good, healthy food, you're telling yourself you're worth it.

Try tasting raw vegetables as you prepare them for cooking – some are more exciting that way. I particularly love raw sugar snap peas. In fact *all* vegetables taste fantastic raw, except for potatoes, which should never be eaten raw, and aubergines (eggplant). Add raw carrots, red (bell) peppers and even fresh peas to salads. They don't have to be limited to tomatoes and limp lettuce.

You need never eat flaccid lettuce again, once you get to know the more unusual greens and leafies that can lift your salad into Michelin territory and detoxify your organs at the same time.

ROMAINE LETTUCE A very crunchy green that has the highest nutrient count of all types of lettuce.

SORREL Pleasantly sour and with a slightly lemony flavour. It's a powerful antioxidant.

SPINACH Most beneficial when eaten raw as baby spinach. Contains many valuable nutrients and is high in iron.

SWISS CHARD From the beet family, Swiss chard has a mild taste and is good with walnuts or pine nuts.

ROCKET (ARUGULA) Peppery and tart, rocket mixes well

with other leaves. High in vitamins A and C, and niacin, iron and phosphorous.

DANDELION GREENS The young leaves have a tangy taste, good for skin disorders, such as eczema. Excellent liver rejuvenator. Rich in calcium, potassium, vitamins A and C. Useful to know about if you happen to be doing a bit of weeding and the shops have closed.

Fruits added to salads make them more interesting. Also, apples, peaches, pears and apricots are wonderful compliments to meats and light cheeses. Salsa up your fish or meat by blending tomatoes or soft fruits, such as peaches or mangoes, with red onion, wine vinegar and a dash of oil.

The rules

- If it grows under the ground – potatoes, carrots, turnips, and so on – start it off in cold water, bring it to the boil and simmer it, covered.
- If it grows above the ground – spinach, cabbage and broccoli, and so on – bring the water to the boil first and cook it without a lid – or better still steam in a colander or steamer.
- Don't ever, ever overcook!

Spuds you like

It's time we unearthed and reconsidered the much maligned, poor old potato. It's still suffering from a bad press as a result of the Atkins-type diets, and is currently a misunderstood, underplayed little root. In fact, potatoes contain strong anti-cancer substances and aid in lowering blood pressure and balancing alkalinity and acidity in the body. They're rich in vitamins, minerals and protein and very high in vitamins A, B and C, and potassium. They contain virtually no fat and have about as many calories as an apple or banana.

Eat the potato skin to get the greatest amount of nutrients from your potato, but not if it's green or has sprouting bits. Peel that part away. To keep potatoes fresh, buy them in small quantities and keep them in a dark place. When exposed to light, potatoes produce a chemical, solanine, which makes them turn green.

> *'I eat potatoes every day. I love potatoes; they're my favourite food, and an important part of my diet. I also enjoy mixing different root vegetables together, such as sweet potatoes, parsnips, swede, beetroot and turnips, and baking or roasting them.'*
>
> **Catherine Hurley**

When you add fat to potatoes, you reduce their nutritional qualities, as well as increasing their fat content, and as most of our potatoes are eaten fried (soaked in fat), mashed (made with butter and cream), baked (served with butter and sour cream) or in a potato salad (with mayonnaise), those of us who are watching our weight tend give potatoes a wide berth.

The way to eat potatoes so you'll never want chips again

These potato 'fans' go with almost anything and taste better than fried, baked or roast potatoes with virtually none of the fat. You can use new or old potatoes, but avoid those big, floury monsters.

METHOD

1 Preheat your oven to 200°C/400°F/Gas 6 and lightly grease a baking tin with olive oil.

2 Put each unpeeled potato in the bowl of a wooden spoon and cut across widthways at 3mm (⅛in) intervals. (The spoon prevents you from cutting right through the potato.)

3 Put the potatoes in the baking tin, give them a fine drizzle of olive oil or spray a fine mist on to them (keep your kitchen oils in sprays so that you use less) and lightly sprinkle with sea salt.

4 Cook for about 1½ hours, depending on their size, until the flesh is soft and the outside gold and crispy. Your shy, retiring spuds should be transformed into beautiful fanned creatures, which taste as delicious as they look.

More ways with potatoes

FOR BAKED POTATOES Try filling with mashed avocado and plain yoghurt (use a fabulous-tasting, creamy, organic yoghurt – there are fat-free versions that taste surprisingly good – not the tasteless, low-fat, globby ones with a blanc-mange-like texture).

FOR MASHED POTATOES Add non-fat plain yoghurt and seasoning instead of butter, then top with chives. If you think this sounds lacking in oomph, remember how you adapted to semi-skimmed (low-fat) milk, and how full-fat (whole) milk now tastes too rich and heavy?

FOR POTATO SALAD Mix half a cup of the above yoghurt with half a cup of low-fat mayonnaise, lemon juice to taste, a tablespoon of chilli sauce and a mashed clove of garlic, or some finely chopped spring onions (scallions).

6

What simply really counts

High carb. Low fat. Low carb. High fat. Eat less calories. Calories don't count. Confusing or what! The real secret of how top models maintain their consistent weight lies in fully understanding the nutritional balance of what they eat, and the physiological dynamics of how they eat – and not in depriving themselves.

Understanding the interaction of the simple food groups is essential for conquering that obsessive, driven, dieting mentality, and helping you to relax and enjoy your food. Poring over the amount of calories, fat, protein, sugar, salt and fibre on labels and worrying about how much of these you should be eating every day is worthless when you don't know what your needs really are.

Learning the strategies to put it all into practice is easy. You don't need a daft 'life coach' in your life, or to learn to love tofu, or go to a place to be weighed and applauded. This chapter will ensure that you'll never fall for misleading and meaningless nutri-babble ever again. This is the definitive crash course in no-bull, nutritional balance.

Things were easier to monitor in the old days. We ate less and better when we had mostly meat and two vegetables on our plates – when we could clearly define the ingredients and they were plainly presented, making the balance of what we were eating easier to assess. Now we have the most stunning, exciting fusion of fabulous world cuisines at our fingertips, but this great variety has also been our downfall. It encourages us to overeat as well as being packed with hidden fats and sugar.

Getting back to basics

First, the basic nutrients: carbohydrates, proteins, fats and water. These are the building blocks for a good diet. By choosing the healthiest forms of each of these nutrients and eating them in the proper balance, your body will perform at its optimum level. Sticking to regular simple meals that contain a starch element, a portion of protein and some vegetables takes away all the stress of counting calories and fat content, and eliminates snacking. But even when you don't have time to prepare or choose simple meals, or sometimes want more exotic food, it's still possible to be aware and in control of how to build up a healthy meal from the basic food groups. For example, if you're hoping to lose a few pounds, you should aim to eat around 1,000 calories a day. If you down a cappuccino and a chocolate croissant for breakfast (390 calories), scoff some banana cake for elevenses

(350 calories) and choose a tuna-mayo baguette for lunch (500 calories), you've blown your day's intake already.

It's the same for fat. Your aim (on a 1,000 calorie diet) is 40g (1½oz) a day, but two slices of deep-pan pizza is double that amount in one hit!

Daily requirements for a sedentary woman

	To maintain weight	To lose weight
Calories	1,900 (kcals)	1,000 (kcals)
Protein	45g (1¾oz)	45g (1¾oz)
Fat	70g (2¾oz)	40g (1½oz)
Saturated fat	20g (¾oz)	15g (½oz)
Sugar	50g (2oz)	25g (1oz)
Salt	6g (⅛oz)	6g (⅛oz)
Fibre (minimum)	18g (⅝oz)	18g (⅝oz)

The facts about calories

Many women are obsessed with calories without knowing what they really are.

Just as electrical energy is measured in watts, the energy we get from food and drink, which powers every activity of cell maintenance and growth, is measured in kilocalories, better known as kcals or, simply, calories.

The total number of calories in your food depends on how much fat, protein and carbohydrate it contains. For every gram of fat in a type of food, you get nine calories. For every gram of protein or carbohydrate, you get just four calories. So foods containing a lot of fat tend to be high in calories.

If you're an average shape and you're trying to maintain, not lose, weight, you should be aiming for a total of around 1,900 calories a day; however, height, age and muscle-to-fat ratios play their own roles, so this is only a benchmark figure. If you eat too many calories, your body will turn them into fat stores. For every 3,500 excess calories you eat, 450g (1lb) of body fat is stored. Eat 3,500 less calories than you need and 450g (1lb) of fat is burned. Most women can lose 900g (2lb) of fat each week by dropping their calorie intake to about 1,000–1,200 a day.

In the endless protein versus carbs debate, a recent study tested two very different diets: one low in carbohydrates and very high in fat, the other high in carbs and low in fat. Both diets totalled 1,000 calories a day. When the two groups of volunteers stepped on the scales after six weeks all of them had lost nearly the same amount of weight and body fat. High fat, low fat, high protein, low protein – none of it made a bit of difference on the scales. What mattered was calorie intake. The key to losing weight is as simple as that.

- Check the amount of calories in a prepared meal by the serving, not per 100g (4oz).
- Don't confuse kcals with kjs, which is short for kilojoules, the metric version for measuring energy in foods. There are 4.2 kilojoules in every calorie.

How different foods affect you

Protein-rich foods – meat, fish, eggs, milk, tofu, pulses, cheese and so on – are filling and will satisfy your hunger for a longer period of time than any other food group. After digesting a small amount of protein your brain sends very clear signals that you're now full up. That's why you can't eat two whole chickens in one go.

Sceptics of the Atkins diet are now suggesting that it is this ability of protein to curb hunger pangs and slightly increase your metabolic rate that is the real reason its devotees lose weight, not Dr Atkins's 'unique discovery', ketosis. Some protein contains the amino acid tryptophan, which encourages your brain to produce the feelgood chemical serotonin. Starchy, carb-rich foods raise serotonin levels, which is why you tend to crave sweet, stodgy and filling carbohydrate food when you're feeling fraught. After a while, when the increased production of serotonin kicks in, you feel your mood lifting. (The anti-depressant drug, Prozac, works by increasing the amount of serotonin in the brain.) If, though, you choose simple carbohydrates containing white flour and refined sugar, hoping for the same quick lift, you'll be disappointed. These foods induce an over-production of insulin, which ensures the energy surge is short lived.

The worst combination of food you can put into your body, as far as your health, well-being and weight are concerned, is fat and sugar – and you know which foods contain these.

Your daily needs

Each day you need to consume adequate amounts of protein, fat, carbohydrate and fibre so that your body will function healthily.

Protein

This is the vital nutrient for the growth and repair of body cells. As well as filling you up, it keeps your metabolism working at its ultimate level. Protein is only one source of calories in your diet, but because gram for gram (ounce for ounce), it supplies half the calories that fat does, foods rich in lean protein – lean meat, white fish and chicken (without the skin) – tend to be quite low in calories. Obviously, the amount of protein you get in a simple serving of protein-rich foods, such as grilled chicken breast, is always going to be higher than the figure on a packet of a ready-prepared dish that contains more than just chicken.

The recommended daily protein intake is 10–15 per cent of total calories, but it's now generally agreed by nutritionists (although not advisable in the long term) that the appetite-suppressing advantages of protein can be safely gained if protein provides up to 25 per cent of daily calories, which works out as a daily protein intake of 400 calories on a diet of 1,200 calories.

To ensure you are getting protein without the fat:

- Go for trimmed, lean red meat and chicken or fish without batter, breadcrumbs or fatty skin.

- Use low-fat cooking methods: grill (broil), bake or roast on a rack; poach; stir-fry or chargrill.

- Brown meat in its own juices.

- Boil, poach or 'fry' eggs in a non-stick pan without added oil.

- Don't eat red meat more than twice a week

Fat

Your body needs fat – really. In fact, fat is the most concentrated source of energy available to the body and provides warmth and healthy bones, eyes and hair. But, after you reach two years old, your body needs only small amounts of fat – much less than is eaten in the average diet. Your diet should not contain more than 30 per cent fat, made up of polyunsaturated and monounsaturated fats.

There are good and bad fats – some toxic, some neutral and some essential to good health. Most people eat too much of the wrong kind. There are three types – saturated, polyunsaturated and monounsaturated, which are based on the number of hydrogen atoms in the chemical structure of a given molecule of fatty acid.

> *TIP* Saturated animal fat is changed when animals are not allowed to eat grass. Grain-fed animals raised without the opportunity to walk round all day produce fat that is deficient in the essential fatty acid omega-3, which is the fat essential for producing the feelgood brain chemical, serotonin. So choosing free-range animal products will always be your healthiest choice.

SATURATED is the fat found in animal products, including eggs and dairy items such as full-fat (whole) milk, cream, cheese and fatty meats like beef, veal, lamb, pork and ham. The fat marbling you see in beef and pork is composed of saturated fat. Some vegetable products, including coconut oil and palm kernel oil are also high in saturates.

The liver uses saturated fats to manufacture cholesterol. So an excessive intake of saturated fats can raise your blood cholesterol level. Huge amounts of bad saturated fats are usually found in processed foods, such as sausages, pies and many cakes, biscuits, savoury snacks and all deep-fried foods and margarine. These hydrogenated (hardened) fats are sometimes called trans fats. They are created when liquid vegetable oils are treated at high temperatures, which changes the unsaturated fat to a solid saturated form, and hydrogenation occurs. Adding hydrogen to fats extends a product's shelf life, but when an oil or fat can't go rancid on the shelf it means your stomach can't digest it either. When you eat these toxic bad fats, your body doesn't recognise them and is unable to process them. They also interfere with the body's ability to process good fats efficiently.

Whereas good fats, such as omega-3s, help to send messages between the junctions of nerve cells in the brain, trans fats invade these junctions, blocking nerve transmissions. If you've been overdoing the trans fats, it's a good idea to use the brain cells you have left to start making smarter choices on the fat front. The daily recommended maximum intake of saturated fat for women is 20g (¾oz), so make sure you check all food labels with this figure in mind.

Oil rules

- Buy cold-pressed (unrefined) oils.
- Avoid hardened oils (hydrogenated), such as margarines.
- Never reuse oil that has been used for frying.
- Keep all oils in a cool, dark cupboard.
- Never consume oil that smells rancid.
- Olive oil maintains a longer shelf life than most oils.
- Don't let oils heat to smoking.
- To sauté or stir-fry, use 30ml (2 tbsp) of water in the oil.
- Best oils are olive, walnut, sesame, flaxseed, almond and avocado.
- Worst oils are coconut, peanut, palm, palm kernel and cottonseed.

POLYUNSATURATED fatty acids have two families: omega-6 and omega-3. Both of these are essential for your brain development. Omega-6s are found in corn, nuts, seeds, soya and sunflower oil. The best source of omega-3s is fish from cold, deep waters, but they're also found in liver, eggs, seafood and the following oils: cod liver, flax, wheatgerm and sesame, walnut, rapeseed and omega-3 enriched foods. Because we get plenty of omega-6 fats from spreads, oils and processed foods, it's best to focus your intake on foods and oils high in omega-3s.

MONOUNSATURATED fatty acids (olive oil, avocados, nuts) are also the good guys because they can actually lower your blood cholesterol level. All three types of fat supply the same amount of calories, but recent research shows that the body metabolises plant-based fats more rapidly than animal fats. So the fat calories derived from seeds, nuts, olive oil and oily fish are burned more quickly in your body than the same number of fat calories from cream.

Watch out for

aerosol whipped cream	luncheon meats
bacon	mayonnaise
butter	offal
chocolate	packaged cakes
coconut	pastries
creamy dressings	peanut butter
fried foods	poultry skin
full-fat (whole) milk	processed cereals
hamburgers	salami
hot dogs	sausages
margarine	smoked meats
ice cream	soft cheese
lard (white cooking fat)	

Carbohydrates

These supply your body with energy and come in two types: complex and simple.

COMPLEX carbohydrates are found in fresh vegetables, fresh fruits, beans and natural whole grains, and provide dietary fibre. They have only one-third of the calories found in fats and simple carbohydrates. A constant flow of energy is supplied from complex carbs, rather than the short-lived energy bursts from simple carbs.

All whole grains, such as corn, oats and rice (except wheat), help reduce fat in the body, but when they're refined they're stripped of bran, the outer part of the grain, and the germ, which leaves them devoid of nutritional value.

SIMPLE carbohydrates are found in these processed and refined grains (not whole grains) and all types of sugar. 'Sugars' is an all-encompassing description that includes not just sucrose (the technical name for the white stuff in our sugar bowls) but sugars that are found naturally in fruit (fructose) and milk (lactose).

To avoid the high energy and fatigue cycle of unregulated blood sugar resulting from eating sugar, top models eat a diet high in the complex carbs and avoid as many refined, processed foods as they can, and most forms of sugars – they contain no valuable nutrients or fibre. This is not just a method to reduce or maintain weight, but a credo to be followed for basic good health.

TIP Apart from the unrefined sugars in fruit fructose and lactose from milk – which are better for you because they avoid sugar rushes and energy highs and lows by being absorbed slowly – it's best, when reading food labels, to avoid those foods that contain ingredients ending with '-ose'.

As well as looking out for glucose, sucrose, dextrose, maltose – all packed with sugar – watch out for hydrolysed starch, brown sugar, maple syrup, blackstrap molasses, golden syrup, honey and treacle. Apart from being found in biscuits, cakes, chocolates, sweets, jams, ice creams, and so on, you'll also find sugar in mayonnaise, tomato ketchup, cereals, drinks, canned fruit, baked beans and even stock cubes.

It's a recognised fact that the food industry capitalises on its knowledge that the sugar/fat combination in snacks and fast foods makes it easy for consumers to overeat. Beat the food companies at their own game by keeping a protein bar, banana or small amount of dried fruit, such as raisins and apricots, in your bag so that you're not tempted by their products.

'I believe in spiral eating — that if you eat sugar, your body will then crave it. If I want a yummy but nutritious snack, I make a chocolate protein shake with rice milk.'

Elle Macpherson

Some artificial sweeteners used in moderation are fine. Cakes and sweets made for diabetics taste exactly the same as the real thing but are sweetened with sorbitol instead of sugar, so they won't produce an over-secretion of insulin that makes you want more and more. Eating normal sugars in moderate quantities is a different matter from eating large amounts of refined sugar. Fructose in a piece of fruit, or lactose in a portion of milk pudding, is not likely to make you fat.

The glycaemic index

To complicate the carbohydrate issue further (no wonder they're called complex) there's a newish way of regulating them called the glycaemic index (GI), on which several recent diet books have been based. This rates a food's GI in terms of its effect on blood glucose levels, but it's just more stuff to think about, and is mostly based on the common sense factor that foods with the highest GI are mainly processed, refined carbs, while vegetables and foods which are densest in nutrients happen to be low GI.

Around 60 per cent of your total daily calories should come from carbohydrates. If much of your diet consists of healthy complex carbohydrates, you should easily consume the recommended daily minimum of 18g (5/8oz) of fibre.

Fibre

This helps to remove fat from the colon wall, and unwanted metals and toxins from our bodies. It's hard to have too much fibre – vegetarians often eat three times this amount. Getting up to 18g (⅝oz) is worth the effort. It keeps your colon in good condition, cuts back the risk of constipation and haemorrhoids, and helps lower blood cholesterol levels. Foods naturally rich in fibre include rye and multigrain bread, oats, high-fibre cereals, pulses, such as red kidney beans, brown rice, nuts, seeds, fruit and vegetables.

Salt

Too much salt raises your blood pressure, which ups your chances of having a stroke. Your daily intake should be under 6g (⅛oz). Some labels list the salt content as sodium, but note that the two are measured differently. To convert the amount of sodium to salt, multiply by 2.5 (6g (⅛oz) of salt a day is roughly the same as 2.5g (⅒oz) of sodium).

Salt cravings are usually a learned response, a habit, unlike sugar cravings, which might be physiological. The more salt you eat, the more you want. Checking labels and choosing low-salt foods is important for controlling your intake. Around two-thirds of the salt we eat comes from processed foods, such as canned soups, meat products, breakfast cereals, bread and savoury snacks. The salt in a packet of crisps has doubled since 1978, and a single-portion 'ready meal', such as chicken korma, contains well over half the recommended daily salt intake.

All supermodels know that too much salt causes you to hang on to excess water in your body, which can lead to swollen ankles and other classic symptoms of bloating and water retention. If you lower your total daily intake of salt still further to 3g (¹⁄₁₆oz) a day, you can shed about 1.5 litres (2½ pints) of excess water, which translates into weight loss on the scales of 1.3kg (3lb).

TIP ■ Choose potassium-rich bananas, potatoes, garlic and dried fruit, as well as your daily intake of water, to help your body eliminate excess salt.
■ Use sea salt in cooking – a little goes a long way.
■ Taste the food on your plate first before reaching for the salt.

Portion sizes

Each day it's advisable to eat around five servings of carbohydrate, two of protein, five of vegetables/fruit and two of dairy. Here's an idea of what you get for each serving:

CARBOHYDRATE 100g (4oz) potatoes, or 125g (4½oz) cooked pasta/rice (the size of your fist), or one 25g (1oz) slice of bread, or half a 60g (2¼oz) roll, or half a 90g (3½oz) pitta bread, or one crumpet, or one 5cm (2in) chunk of French bread, or a quarter of a naan bread, or a 40g (1½oz) serving of breakfast cereal.

PROTEIN 100g (4oz) lean meat, chicken, fish or game (the size of a deck of cards), or one egg, or 125g (4½oz) cooked pulses or 150g (5oz) tofu.

VEGETABLES/FRUIT 80g (3¾oz) of any vegetable or fruit. A five-a-day portion could be a medium apple or banana, a bowl of mixed salad, half a grapefruit, a handful of grapes, a cupped handful of vegetables (raw, cooked, frozen or canned), a slice of melon, ten radishes, three sticks of celery or 20 raspberries.

DAIRY 250ml (8fl oz) skimmed or soya milk, or 200g (7oz) low-fat yoghurt, or 25g (1oz) reduced-fat cheddar, or 40g (1½oz) goat's cheese.

What's your food fix?

Those are the food facts; now discover your food fix by answering the questions below.

1. Which one of the following do you do the most often:

   a) Overeat when tense and nervous?

   b) Need an afternoon snack to keep going?

   c) Enjoy buttered toast for the butter more than the toast?

   d) Often eat pasta for supper because it's comforting?

2. When eating out, which one of the following are you most likely to do:

   a) Add salt to your food before tasting?

   b) Leave room for the pudding?

   c) Choose the creamiest foods?

   d) Reach for the bread basket?

3. Feeling peckish? Which one of the following are you most likely to do?

   a) Enjoy something sweet but prefer alternate sweet and salty snacks?

    b) Go for ice cream?

    c) Grab some cheese or peanut butter?

    d) Hit on a bagel and don't care what goes in it?

4. How do you prefer your toast:

    a) With Marmite?

    b) With jam?

    c) With melted butter?

    d) With anything – you're not fussy?

5. Do you mostly:

    a) Rarely show interest in puddings?

    b) Fret if forced to skip meals?

    c) Hate the taste of low-fat foods?

    d) Start the day with toast and cereal?

6. You're at a petrol station. There's a long drive ahead and you're hungry. Do you pick up:

    a) Crisps?

    b) Chocolate or sweets?

    c) Sausage roll?

    d) Sandwich?

IF YOU SCORED MOSTLY As: it's time to shake the salt habit. Stop adding so much salt to your cooking and food –

add herbs and spices instead. Wine tastes great in sauces, so does mustard. You're suffering from dietary stress, which your body is not coping with efficiently, and is drawing you into a cycle of craving sugar and salt. Don't skip meals, and try to find ways to relax. Try to prepare fresh food but if that's not possible, remember to read labels – the higher up the label the salt is listed the more salt there is in the product. Remember: no more than 6g (⅛oz) a day!

IF YOU SCORED MOSTLY BS: can't resist a sugar fix as the day goes on, sweetie? Make sure you eat protein with every meal to ensure you give your brain what it needs to make natural mood enhancers, such as serotonin, rather than relying on sugar to give the same effect. Start eating more complex carbs, such as pasta, brown rice, oats and rye, which provide slow-release energy that the body gradually converts to sugar, thus avoiding dramatic blood-sugar surges.

IF YOU SCORED MOSTLY CS: your fix is fat – you crave cheese and other rich foods. Everyone needs fat, but when you crave saturated fats, such as butter and cream, it means your body is unable to differentiate between the bad and good fats, and you're likely to be deficient in omega-3 fatty acids. Eat more oily fish, such as trout, sardines or organic salmon, and replace the saturated fat in the cheese with monounsaturated fats in olives and nuts. Try sprinkling a tablespoon of linseeds on your cereal or salad every day.

IF YOU SCORED MOSTLY DS: You're addicted to starch and find carbs, such as bread and pasta, comforting. Your meals often include little or no protein, and if you feel low in the evenings and lack daylight in winter, you're probably suffering from low serotonin (the brain's feelgood chemical). Eat protein, such as fish, beef, chicken and eggs, with as many meals as possible and always opt for complex carbs rather than refined ones to avoid dramatic surges.

The model way to eat

One-third of your diet should be made up of complex carbs – wholegrain cereals, such as oats, rye, barley, wholemeal (whole-wheat) bread, brown rice, muesli, porridge, pasta, beans and potatoes.

Another third consists of colourful fruit and vegetables: berries, cantaloupe melon, leafy green vegetables and red (bell) peppers, salads, dried fruits, fresh nuts or seeds.

The final third is a bit more complicated. Just imagine it divided into three – two equal parts that make up 80 per cent of the total and a third smaller part that is only 20 per cent. One large part consists of cheese, milk, yoghurt and eggs; the second of meat, fish, poultry or vegetarian proteins. Add healthy fats by drizzling a tablespoon of flaxseed (linseed) or olive oil on to the food. The final 20 per cent represents cream, butter, biscuits, cakes, ice cream, chocolates and other occasional treats.

The fibre in the grains, fruit and vegetables helps ensure a steady supply of energy because it slows the body's absorption of carbohydrates, a key energy source.

The colourful fruits and vegetables give you energy-producing vitamins and minerals. The lean protein and healthy fats found in the flaxseed oil and fatty fish help to keep your brain active. All these foods work synergistically to keep your body at its peak power.

Eating in this way means you automatically get around half your calories from complex carbohydrates, while less than a third come from fat – with the fewest of these from the least healthy saturated fat – and around 12 per cent will come from protein.

TIP Learn to listen to your body – some foods increase your vitality and well-being; others diminish it. Determine which foods are your personal high-energy foods by eating a food you like. Notice your body sensations 45 to 60 minutes later. If you feel clear and energetic, you ate a high-energy food for you. If you don't, you didn't!

Water, water, water

There isn't a supermodel in existence who doesn't start her day with a glass of hot water, best drunk on its own, but sometimes with a few drops of lemon juice. All models consider water to be their essential beauty product. It's the most vital nutrient of all, cleansing the liver, kidneys and digestive system and directly affecting the look and feel of your skin. Without water, life would end in 3–5 days, although we can survive without food for 30–40 days. Fine, but it's often confusing to know how much we should be drinking. We read conflicting data every day: 'Drink two litres a day, at least', 'Eight glasses minimum' (well, how big is the glass?), 'One litre plus a glass for every coffee and …' What are we to believe? No one seems to take body size into account when suggesting these amounts. Surely Kylie Minogue needs less water than Arnold Schwarzenegger? Drinking too much water can do more damage than good – it washes out the minerals and sodium your body needs. The Chinese committed suicide by drinking too much water!

So how much is right for you? The simple way to work out the correct, manageable quantity for your body is by drinking one 250ml (8fl oz) glass of water per 9kg (20lb) of your body weight. Drink before you get thirsty – being thirsty means that you're already dehydrated; check the colour of your urine: the darker the colour, the more dehydrated you are. A light straw colour is the perfect-looking pee.

> **TIP** Often we think we're hungry when actually we're simply thirsty. If you drink sufficient water you'll know that any hunger you feel is really about wanting food.

The permanent accessory of supermodels is not the latest designer handbag, but a small bottle of mineral water. Most of the girls drink Evian – a good choice, rich in minerals, with a distinctive soft, clean taste. Established in

1878, this is a classic, consistent, smart all-rounder. San Pellegrino or Badoit are often their choice in European restaurants. These have a slightly salty taste and a high percentage of calcium and magnesium, so are good for bones. They're naturally carbonated, unlike all other fizzy waters, which are carbonated versions of the original found at source. Easy to drink, these two naturals are not fiercely, falsely effervescent and so don't bloat your tum.

Don't ever believe the hype about expensive mineral waters. A recent release, developed by an Austrian naturalist, and costing 25 times more than the average bottled water, claims to 'remove the negative memories from the water and transfer beneficial energy patterns to it'. Eau dear.

A supermodel trick is to buy cases of handbag-sized bottles (bulk order them on-line from supermarkets and have them delivered free) and dot them around the areas they frequent the most: desk, car, kitchen worktop, next to the stereo, telly and bed. That way, they take a swig whenever they see a bottle and can monitor how many small bottles they drink a day.

The message in your bottle

The convenience of bottled water is a major selling point, but don't be conned into thinking that anything you buy in a bottle is automatically purer and healthier than tap water. Supermarket bottled water could be up to two years old and have a lower mineral content than your own tap water. Two-thirds of what's sold in this country is natural mineral water, which is a legally protected term. To qualify, the water must come from a known and protected source, be bottled at that source and have a consistent mineral analysis – the health-generating properties – with that analysis printed on the label.

Most natural mineral waters and many spring waters have filtered through rocks for millennia before surfacing. This makes 'freshness' a non-issue. A year or two in the bottle makes no odds. Nearly all the other bottled water on sale is spring water, which also comes from an underground source that can be treated to remove impurities and need not be consistent in its mineral composition from bottle to bottle.

NATURAL MINERAL WATER Stringent regulations ensure it's reasonably pure and unpolluted. Most taste good, although they can be expensive. The plastics in bottles (PFCs) can leach into the water and act as hormone disrupters.

SPRING WATER Fairly pure and unpolluted. Taste depends on brand, although they tend to be expensive.

TAP WATER Convenient and cheap. Taste depends on where you live. Can be as pure as mineral water, but can also contain chlorine and other disinfectant chemicals. Needs to be drawn before drinking every morning. If left standing for several hours, lead may have leached into it. Don't drink from bathroom taps if the water doesn't come direct from the mains. Don't drink from hot taps as they can have high copper levels.

FILTERED WATER Many water filters use carbon, and they mainly remove chemicals such as chlorine and ammonia.

The filters need replacing regularly or they can leach bacteria back to the water. Sophisticated systems use reverse osmosis – a system through which only water molecules can pass, resulting in water resembling rainwater. Great taste, pollution free, no plastic bottles. Expensive outlay initially, but worth the cost long term.

7

The food models love

There's nothing like taste and smell to roll back times and places for us – food is the trigger for our memories. Favourite tastes make us feel safe and loved. It's why we often eat too many things we shouldn't, because it makes us think of home. I'm not talking post-hangover carb-fest here, but about the food that was cooked for you as a child, the manner of eating, the associations of family, heritage and that sense of belonging that comes from every mouthful of food we feel familiar with. I still feel a wave of nostalgia whenever I eat my favourite childhood meal of scrambled eggs on buttery toast. No one could quite cook them like my late, wonderful mum, especially when followed by some butterscotch instant whip decorated with mandarin orange segments and presented to me on a racing-green wooden tray with reassuring side panels.

Mum had a great way with trays. It was how she made mealtime sense out of the chaotic ebb and flow of feeding endless people at different times. When my father died and money was tight, she took in lodgers – or PGs (paying guests) as she preferred to call them. She styled each tray to suit its recipient: with the first summer rose from the garden; a newspaper cutting relating to a subject she knew you were passionate about; some funny photograph taken by one of her students (she was the local drama college bursar). My mother hated cooking, but her presentation was legendary, making a Fray Bentos meat pie with peas look Michelin-worthy.

She was the latte of human kindness, and it's no surprise that in a recent poll it was rice pudding, ice cream and mashed potatoes that topped the list of Brits' favourite comfort foods, all nice and creamy – just like mother's milk. Told we can't have these oral security blankets any more, we eventually rebel. Which is why diets don't work. Models know this only too well and that's why they use 'flexible restraint' rather than 'rigid restraint' (strict, unbending dietary rules) to stay on a healthy eating course.

'I love to eat white fish when I'm out — my favourite is halibut. I don't cook fish at home because I don't really like handling it, but I love to eat it in restaurants. I'm also mad about fresh cream cakes. That's my real comfort food. I like sweets now and then — wine gums preferably.'

Catherine Hurley

Flexible restraint means sometimes eating your favourite comfort foods or having an exotic meal out, while mainly following a healthy-eating routine. Most models stick to the 80/20 ratio, where 80 per cent of what they eat is highly nutritious and 20 per cent is a desired treat.

When Kate Moss flew back from Stella McCartney's wedding, where the reception served vegetarian food, she was seen tucking in to a Thai duck salad with bread rolls and two large wedges of chocolate cake on board her flight. Had she been suffering too much rigid 'vegetarian' restraint?

Having a nutrient-packed diet means you can handle a moderate amount of unhealthy treats. But if you're under-weight or overweight, or drinking too much alcohol or coffee, the toxic load will be too great to eat any junk. Perversely, that's when you'll crave it most. The key to using flexible restraint successfully lies in never cheating on the deal you make with yourself. It means not snacking randomly between meals and knowing that too many take-aways and pre-prepared food will drain your vitality and add on the pounds. It means making rules that are yours alone: eating less on Tuesday when you overdo it on Monday; cutting out bread after lunch; swapping a whole bar of chocolate for a couple of pieces; learning to drizzle things in oil or cream instead of drowning them; having that huge hunk of cheese you craved instead of a meal, not as well as. Realising that if you eat huge dinners every night with all the trimmings, you'll get fat.

Supermodels' favourite comfort foods

....

'I drink some full-fat milk, which I often boil first and drink with some brown sugar.'

Alek Wek

'A cup of tea and toast with Marmite when I get up, while reading the newspapers.'

Claudia Schiffer

'Salty liquorice — all Danish people love it. I carry bags of it around for me and my friends.'

Helena Christensen

'I eat a couple of pieces of organic dark chocolate every day.'

Jerry Hall

Models see foods as they really are. They know you can't be slim and eat chocolate brownies all the time but you can have them as treats. It's up to you to decide whether you're willing to sacrifice being energetic, happy, self-confident, slim and more attractive for the constant but fleeting momentary taste of something sweet.

It's all about thinking 'slim'; when eating food is just another part of your life, like work, friends and shopping, rather than thinking 'fat', which is when you eat diet products, are always on a diet and think about food constantly.

Say cheese

Photographer and supermodel Helena Christensen's favourite shop in the world is a cheese store in Paris. She loves the stuff. When you eat cheese in moderation (a healthy portion size is 25g (1oz) or a matchbox-sized chunk) it provides a boost of essential nutrients including protein, vitamin D and zinc as well as calcium, which are essential for bones. Check out the nutritional values of the ones you enjoy:

BRIE Lower levels of fat than Cheddar or Stilton and a good quantity of calcium.

CAMEMBERT A third less fat and a quarter fewer calories than hard cheeses. High in folic acid, although avoid if pregnant, as it's mould-ripened, like Brie.

COTTAGE CHEESE The only truly low-fat cheese, but it also has a low calcium content, which reduces its nutritional rating compared to other cheeses.

CHEDDAR One of the highest-fat cheeses, but a good source of calcium and zinc.

CREAM CHEESE The unhealthiest cheese, as it's close to 50 per cent pure fat and has only a fraction of the calcium content of many hard cheeses.

EDAM Contains a medium amount of fat, is rich in calcium, but high in salt.

EMMENTHAL/GRUYÈRE Very high protein, calcium and

zinc content (essential for healthy skin, reproduction and immune system) though a higher fat ratio than edam.

FETA Made with sheep's milk, it has a moderate amount of calcium and fewer calories than half-fat Cheddar. A better source of vitamin D than cow's milk cheese, but it is also the saltiest.

GOAT'S CHEESE Low in calories and richer in vitamin D (an important bone-strengthener) compared with cow's milk cheeses, although not a great source of calcium or zinc.

HALF-FAT CHEDDAR Higher in protein, calcium and zinc than normal Cheddar, but a bit lower in vitamins A and D.

PROCESSED CHEESE SLICES Rich in calcium, lower in saturated fats than unprocessed cheese. Gets its 'plastic appeal' from added milk proteins, modified starch, preservatives and emulsifiers.

MOZZARELLA A medium-fat cheese which can be disproportionately high in unhealthy saturates. Good calcium content.

PARMESAN Extremely high in calcium. This is the best cheese for zinc but it is high in salt.

RICOTTA Fairly low in fat and salt and contains low to medium amounts of calcium.

STILTON Similar to Cheddar in fat and calories, but has a much lower calcium content. It is high in folic acid, like all blue-veined cheese, but not suitable for pregnant woman as it carries a listeria warning because of the mould.

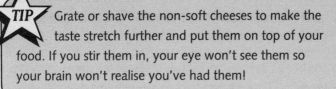

TIP Grate or shave the non-soft cheeses to make the taste stretch further and put them on top of your food. If you stir them in, your eye won't see them so your brain won't realise you've had them!

Game on

Chicken and turkey are everyone's favourites because they're lean, clean and easy to eat, but a tad boring, pretty tasteless and yawningly predictable unless they're jazzed up with spices and sauces or free-range. Game birds (partridge, quail, pheasant and grouse), on the other hand, are naturally organic, because they roam happy and free. They're rich in healthy protein and packed with the full range of B vitamins, iron and zinc, and are extremely low in saturated fat.

The ultimate comfort food is a roast pheasant with all the trimmings. It's as easy as roasting a chicken, and next day you can eat the leftover bits, which make a mind-blowingly delicious salad. For a superb weekend treat for two, you'll need a pheasant each if you want to make the following roast and the salad on consecutive days. The recipes are for one person.

Incredibly easy roast pheasant

METHOD

1   Preheat the oven to 200°C/400°F/Gas 6. Brush an oven-ready large, but young, pheasant with olive oil, salt and

pepper and place it in a roasting pan. Cover it with streaky bacon rashers. Cook in the oven for 1 hour or until tender. Lift on to a platter.

2   For the gravy, reserve 15ml (1 tbsp) of the juices from the tin, add 175ml (6fl oz) chicken stock (a low-salt cube is fine), 15ml (1 tbsp) redcurrant jelly and bring to the boil. Stir until it's lightly thickened.

3   Serve the breasts of the pheasant with Brussels sprouts, the crispy bacon bits, fan potatoes (see page 81) and packet bread sauce made with skimmed milk. This is comfort food without the damage.

Cold pheasant salad

This is a robust salad with warm redcurrant and balsamic vinegar dressing.

METHOD

1   Tear the leftover pheasant pieces into shreds and put in a serving bowl with a trimmed and sliced fennel bulb, the separated leaves of two small heads of chicory and 100g (4oz) of walnut halves.

2   For the dressing, heat 45ml (3 tbsp) redcurrant jelly until it's melted and stir in 30ml (2 tbsp) of balsamic vinegar. Lower the heat and whisk in 5ml (1 tsp) Dijon mustard, then 15ml (1 tbsp) sunflower oil. Remove from the heat, season and add the juice of half a lemon. Pour on to salad leaves and pheasant pieces, toss well and serve at once.

Fishes for dishes

Most models prefer eating fish to meat. We all know the benefits of eating fish, but with recent scares about farmed salmon and the high levels of mercury in swordfish, which are the healthiest options?

COD Low in fat and calories, high in iodine and vitamin B_{12}. As a white fish, it has low quantities of omega-3s and only a trace of vitamin D.

HADDOCK Rich in iodine with more than double the amount found in cod. Also higher in calcium and iron than cod . One fillet provides a day's supply of vitamin B_{12}.

KIPPERS High in salt, but richer in vitamins D and B_{12} than virtually any other food. Our bodies can store supplies of these vitamins for later use, which means just one large kipper fillet every one or two weeks is enough to supply all we require.

MACKEREL The richest source of omega-3 oils, apart from Norwegian sardines. Also rich in vitamins B_{12}, D and iodine. Choose fresh, not high-salt smoked.

MONKFISH Like other white fish, monkfish is low in calories and fat, and also low in beneficial omega-3s. However, it has good levels of vitamin B_{12} and iodine.

SARDINES – THE WINNER A fabulous source of omega-3s and, eaten with the bones, a very rich source of minerals. A serving of four sardines provides more than half the day's supply of calcium, a third of iron, and a tenth of zinc. However, the salt content in canned sardines is high.

Fish tips

- Poached fish will be firmer and whiter if you add a dash of lemon juice to the liquid.
- Try poaching fish in white wine – it gives it a new dimension.
- Thaw frozen fish in milk. The milk draws out the frozen taste and provides a fresh-caught flavour.
- If your fish smells fishy, the fish oils are becoming rancid. Unless you live in a coastal area, or have a great fishmonger nearby, your best bet is frozen fish – it's frozen within hours of being caught, whereas fresh is often transported for days before reaching the market.

SALMON Rich in omega-3 oils and an excellent source of vitamin B_{12}. However, it is advisable to limit non-organic consumption to one portion a week because of possible contamination with dioxins and other pollutants. Smoked salmon retains all the beneficial omega-3 oils but an average portion contains half the daily supply of salt.

SHELLFISH A reasonable source of iodine and selenium. Prawns and mussels supply more calcium gram per gram (ounce per ounce) than milk, and cockles are a rich source of iron.

SWORDFISH Can contain high levels of mercury so should not be eaten too often. Mercury can harm the nervous system of an unborn child so pregnant women should avoid it. Mercury content aside, it's low fat, high protein, rich in vitamin B_{12} and iodine.

TUNA Canned oily fish is usually as healthy as fresh, but tuna is the exception: the canning process allows the omega-3 oils to leach away. However, a serving of either canned or fresh tuna provides a day's supply of vitamin D and selenium.

WHITEBAIT These fish are eaten whole with bones, which means they provide a day's supply of calcium in a 100g (4oz) serving, and a third more iron than the same weight of rump steak. However, they are usually fried, which makes them high in calories and fat.

Beyond the shell

We don't always want our protein in the form of meat and fish, and eggs are the perfect answer: they're low in calories and high in nutrients. The tastiest eggs are organic and free-range (which means their yolks are vivid yellow), so make these your first choice.

> **TIP** To tell if an egg is fresh, place it in a bowl of cold water. If it lies flat on the bottom it's very fresh; if it stands upright with the egg still touching the bottom it's okay; but if it floats, chuck it out.

If you can't locate those beauties, go for simply organic. Then choose free-range or (lower down the scale) barn-reared and, finally, there are battery cage, which should be avoided at all costs. Eggs are so inexpensive it's worth paying every penny to buy the best.

How to make the perfect omelette ...

... and not a leathery old tosser:

1. Buy yourself a non-stick omelette pan.
2. Don't add water, milk or cream – they thin out the mixture and the eggs lose their viscosity.
3. Use butter, not oil.
4. Make sure the eggs are not over-beaten when added.
5. Keep the eggs moving with a fork, similar to making scrambled eggs.
6. When the omelette's the right consistency for you, leave it for 30 seconds to set the base.
7. Roll, don't fold, to retain the fluffy texture.

Yo, yoghurt!

This is a supreme superfood with enormous healthy benefits, yet it's cosy and so simple – basically milk with friendly bacteria added. These bacteria produce an enzyme that attacks the natural milk sugar, lactose, producing lactic acid that curdles the milk and gives yoghurt its tart taste.

Packed with protein, calcium, potassium, phosphorus, vitamins B_6, B_{12}, and A and D, and with lactobacillus acidophilus and other friendly bacteria that aid digestion. Frankly, yoghurt protects you from just about everything.

An American study has found that dieters who include a fat-free yoghurt as part of their diet plan lose significantly more weight than those who simply cut calories. The calcium helps to speed up the weight-loss process. It triggers the body to burn more fat and reduce the amount of new fat the body makes. But not all yoghurts are equal. In the manufacture of cheap yoghurt, high-speed machinery pumps the yoghurt along miles of pipes. This breaks its delicate structure which traditionally comes from the natural thickening associated with the incubation of bacteria. So gums are added at the beginning of the process to make it 'bullet-proof' which gives the product it's blancmange-like texture.

A typical low-fat strawberry yoghurt contains not just yoghurt and strawberries but also modified starch to thicken it and replace the texture of fruit; gelatine, gums or pectin to make it gel; colouring and flavourings; and some form of fructose (corn sugar). A 'strawberry yoghurt' must contain some fruit, a 'strawberry-flavoured yoghurt' has had a brief fling with the fruit, while a 'strawberry-flavour yoghurt' has never even met a strawberry!

Yoghurt that is really good for you should be sugar-free and organic, containing the acidophilus bacteria. Some makers heat it to extend its shelf life, destroying most of the active cultures (friendly bacteria) and therefore the healthy benefits. Be sure the label states 'live' or 'active cultures'. Buy yoghurt that has an expiry date at least ten days ahead. If there is no date, don't buy it.

Some yoghurt culture

There are herdsmen in the Soviet Republic of Georgia and Armenia who live to be more than 120 years old. They eat enthusiastic amounts of yoghurt every day and almost never have any incidence of cancer.

FLAVOURS MODELS FAVOUR

Models buy organic, fat-free plain, thick, creamy delicious yoghurts with plenty of probiotic bacteria to help keep their bodies in balance, and then add sweetness, because ready-bought fruit yoghurts are mostly loaded with sugar. They add:

- French or Spanish sugar-free fruit jam.

- Juice nectar – pear, apricot, peach.

- Apple sauce with a dash of cinnamon and raisins.

- Manuka honey from New Zealand.

- Chopped banana, crushed roasted almonds, clear honey.

TIP When taking antibiotics, wait at least an hour before eating yoghurt or any other dairy product. The calcium in yoghurt and other dairy products may interfere with the drug's actions.

Milking it?

Supermodel Alex Wek loves to drink a glass of milk, but fear not if this doesn't appeal, as milk isn't the best source of calcium: it doesn't contain much magnesium, which is needed to metabolise calcium. Eating a yoghurt a day alongside organic, calcium-fortified soya, goat's or rice milk and a diet rich in seeds and leafy vegetables, *will* give you adequate calcium and magnesium. Here are the different types of milk and their nutritional benefits:

COW'S MILK The most popular is semi-skimmed, which, together with skimmed, contains slightly more calcium than full-fat (whole) milk and less fat.

GOAT'S MILK has a softer curd and smaller fat molecules than cow's milk, making it easier to digest. It is a good choice for those with delicate digestions or stomach ulcers, but can taste a bit 'goaty'.

RICE MILK Like soya milk, it is 100 per cent non-dairy, low in fat and lactose-free. It is a good choice for vegans and those who are lactose intolerant. It is usually fortified with calcium, but has virtually no protein, so you have to get your protein sources elsewhere.

SOYA MILK Low in saturated fat and rich in protein, soya milk is a good choice for those intolerant to cow's milk. Only drink soya milk made from the whole bean and always choose a brand that's calcium-fortified and organic to avoid genetic modification.

Soya benefits

Before you give me the Hypocrite of the Year Award for all my tofu jibes, let me just say that I still hate tofu – how anyone can enjoy eating a food that takes on the taste of whatever you're cooking with it, rather than having its own distinct flavour, is beyond me – but some models love it, and there are other soya products that taste fine.

The fact is the humble soybean is a nutritional giant for women, as it contains isoflavones (natural plant hormones also known as phytoestrogens) that are vital to our health, plus calcium, minerals and vitamins. It's one of the few plants that provides a complete protein source while being low in fat. You need only 25g (1oz) of soya protein a day to enjoy the benefits of the bean.

Asian countries have worshipped soya for centuries, but until recently it was seen here as the sole property of vegetarians, who rely on it as a major protein source.

It has obvious benefits to women – the isoflavones help protect against osteoporosis, and it can help protect against hormone-dependent cancers in the breast and ovaries. It is worth noting, however, that the toxins in soya are not completely removed by boiling but are removed through fermentation. Fermented soya includes shoyu, tamari, miso and tempeh. There's a diverse selection of soya products to choose from in the marketplace:

MISO Soybeans fermented into a meaty paste – good for seasonings.

SOYA MILK Thinner than dairy milk but not bad on cereals and muesli. Not great in tea or coffee.

SOYA YOGHURTS These taste good and, being dairy-free, are lactose-free. Definitely worth trying.

TAMARI A naturally aged and fermented soy sauce. This is a great product. Really!

TOFU Bean curd. A white, cheese-like texture, bland in taste, which takes on the flavour of any food combined with it. The curdled soya milk is pressed into a cake and sold vacuum-packed in water. Yum. There are two types of tofu: firm and silky. Firm is more versatile; silky is best eaten raw (by someone other than me) or used in soups. But it doesn't stir-fry well. What a surprise.

Keeping it sweet

Who would have thought that the old Jezebel, *chocolate*, has a greater antioxidant capacity than some fruit and vegetables? Well, Jerry Hall for one. Limiting cholesterol and boosting the immune system is just the beginning of its untold talents. Chocolate also contains a fair bit of calcium, iron, vitamins A, B_1, C, D and E, traces of zinc and copper and phenols, which protect against heart disease. It's a major source of magnesium, which is food for the nervous system and a muscle relaxant, one of the reasons we crave it around our period. Eating chocolate up to three times a month enables people to live a year longer than others, claims America's Harvard School of Public Health.

An amino acid contained in chocolate, called phenyl ethylamine, acts as an aphrodisiac and is also useful for banishing hangovers. And, because it melts at 34ºC (93ºF), chocolate will dissolve the instant you pop it into your mouth, speeding up the rate at which all these nutrients are absorbed.

Too good to be true? Almost. Chocolate can be addictive, especially if the type you're eating contains less than 20 per cent cocoa solids and lots of sugar. There's a fine line between embracing these unexpected benefits respectfully, and overdoing it. Carefully does it – a little goes a long way.

- Eat chocolate with, or soon after, a meal when you'll be less tempted to overeat.

- Choose plain chocolate that contains a minimum of 70 per cent cocoa solids or milk chocolate with at least 30 per cent.

- Buy less; buy better-quality chocolate in small bars, rather than boxes.

- To avoid the depressed or stressed-out binge, eat small servings once or twice a week.

- Choose bars with choc chips or choc chunks rather than full-on chocolate.

- Eat dark chocolate – it's higher in antioxidants than milk chocolate.

- Learn how to eat chocolate for its full effect, so that less becomes more. Let it sit in your mouth for a few seconds to release its primary aromas. Then chew it a few times to release the secondary aromas. Then rest it lightly against the roof of your mouth to experience the full range of its flavours and textures and then ... okay, that's enough.

Sweet secrets

....

Ever since I opened my deli, I've been searching the world for the ultimate-tasting sugar-free chocolate; and recently I found it in Belgium – in milk, dark and white chocolate. To celebrate my discovery, I've introduced some sugar-free chocolate praline supermodel lips to my deli. Not only do they taste sublime, but they look sexy and amazing – and are, of course, sugar-free. See my website at the back of the book for mail-order details.

If, however, going anywhere near chocolate is too dangerous for you, but you've a sweet tooth that needs satisfying, I have the perfect answer. Amazake is a wonderful Japanese product that tastes so interestingly good. It's a rich, creamy dessert, with no added sweeteners or dairy ingredients, made according to a traditional Oriental recipe, by cooking whole millet grains and adding a special culture called koji. The koji reduces the starches in the grain into their own sugars, without depleting the grain of its wholesome goodness, resulting in a nutritious, naturally sweet pudding that's easily digested and gluten-free. It can be served straight from the jar as a hot or cold dessert or topping.

Every model who shops at the deli buys one of these 'sweet secrets' – except for Elizabeth Hurley, who prefers our Manuka honey, a delicious dark New Zealand honey, which is brilliant for strengthening the immune system.

Also popular with models are the French and Spanish jams made from old recipes, which contain no sugar. The fruit is slow-cooked in grape juice to give it a natural sweetness and fruity flavour. They're great for mixing with plain yoghurts. Liquorice devotees love the sugar-free, fat-free liquorice coins I found on a recent trip to Holland, not only because they taste completely delicious, but also because they're good laxatives.

These items are available by mail order from my website if you have difficulty sourcing them. Amazake is the generic name so can be found worldwide.

Foods that match

Claudia Schiffer loves toast with Marmite, which is the perfect match of two foods. It's not always what you eat, but what you eat with what, that counts. Some foods work together better than others to enhance the absorption of nutrients.

CHEESE AND RED WINE The fat and milk proteins in cheese line the stomach to slow down alcohol release into the blood, while the flavonoids in red wine stimulate calcium absorption. These compounds also work as antioxidants in the blood, protecting arteries from the build-up of fatty deposits.

FISH OR MEAT WITH SALAD Concentrated protein, such as fish and meat, need a lot of stomach acid and three hours to be absorbed. It's even more work if you combine it with other hard-to-digest-foods, such as cheese, or carbo-hydrates, such as potatoes. Occasionally eating fish or meat with only a salad enables your stomach to focus on digesting protein only, allowing your body to benefit from the proteins, iron and vitamins it contains.

FRUITS AND NUTS WITH MUESLI Vitamin C and substances called flavonoids in fruit work together to enhance the absorption of vitamin E, calcium and iron found in seeds and nuts. If you add live yoghurt, the beneficial bacteria enhance the absorption of B vitamins from the muesli and synthesise vitamin K in the gut.

WHOLEGRAIN BREAD WITH MARMITE Whole grains and yeast extracts, such as Marmite, are one of the richest sources of B vitamins and chromium. These nutrients boost energy and brain function and help control the breakdown of fat. The B vitamins in whole grains will encourage the absorption of those in Marmite.

Sixteen nutrient-packed tips

1. Use potatoes with the skins on, even for potato salad.
2. Use more stems and leaves, such as celery.
3. Eat white foods (except for cauliflower) in small quantities. Colour equals vitamin content.
4. Use sweet potatoes more frequently – they're pounding with nutrients.
5. Avoid stale food. Buy the freshest food possible.
6. Eat raw fruit and vegetables twice a day.
7. Use a cooking method, such as steaming, that minimises vitamin and mineral loss.
8. Don't combine fresh fruits with other food if possible; eat fruit alone.

9. Don't use aluminium pans.
10. Use very little water when steaming vegetables.
11. Avoid fried and processed foods.
12. Don't fry foods in hydrogenated oils.
13. Use edible seaweed in soups and casseroles – it's the richest source of minerals.
14. Wash all melons before cutting to avoid transferring bacteria from the skin on to the flesh. Don't juice the rind.
15. Don't use cans if they bulge or the top isn't tight.
16. Use foods in their natural state as much as possible.

All-time supermodel superfoods

ALMOND The king of nuts. High in potassium, magnesium, phosphorus and protein. Not all the fat, and therefore the calories, of almonds is absorbed – a non-fattening characteristic that also occurs with pecans. Chestnuts have the lowest fat content.

AVOCADO Combats fatigue and nerves from the inside, perks up facial skin from the outside. Contains *all* the antioxidant vitamins and is packed with minerals.

BLUEBERRY A great blood cleanser, rich in vitamins C and E, which feed the brain, and nutrients that alleviate eye strain. All berries are superbly good for you.

CANTALOUPE MELON Provides more vitamins A (beta-carotene) and C than most other fruits. High in potassium. It is an excellent cleanser and rehydrator. Should be eaten on its own for maximum benefit.

CHICKEN, TURKEY AND GAME BIRDS The healthiest meat, low in fat and high in protein. Buy organic poultry and avoid frozen, imported birds, which may contain bulking agents.

CHOCOLATE Because most supermodels can't imagine life without it!

GARLIC AND GINGER Nature's own antibiotics. They're antibacterial, antiseptic, antiviral, and decongestant. They also lower cholesterol, and contain calcium, phosphorus and potassium. Use in stir-fries.

GREEN TEA Contains supernutrients, called satechins, which help the liver break down fat. This, combined with the ability of satechins to boost metabolism, suggests that green tea helps weight loss. Also contains the EGCG flavonoid, which is 100 times more powerful as an antioxidant than vitamin C.

LINSEEDS These seeds have brilliant scouring powers. Sprinkle a tablespoonful each day on your cereal or salad. Eat only raw seeds and those in tightly sealed bags, as roasted seeds go off when exposed to light and air.

OATS The protein content is easily assimilated and helps neutralise excess cholesterol. Contains high amounts of calcium, iodine, magnesium, iron and the major vitamins.

OYSTERS For cardiovascular, immune and sexual functions. Very high in zinc which helps the skin to maintain its collegen supply and also contains vitamin A, vitamin B$_{12}$, vitamin C and iron. They are temperamental little beasts (being sexy, raw and quivering) so don't like competing with vodka or any other spirit.

PAPAYA Great detoxifier and excellent for aiding digestion. Soothes intestinal inflammation and gas. Contains calcium, magnesium, potassium, vitamin C and betacarotene.

SEA VEGETABLES A power-packed supermodel essential for growing strong nails, hair, bones and teeth. Kelp is the most popular variety, and granulated kelp is a good substitute for salt, used daily in your diet.

TOMATOES A great natural source of supernutrients, including lycopene, which protects against heart disease and cancer.

SWEET POTATOES Fabulously detoxifying – they bind to heavy-metal deposits and remove them from the body. Good for poor circulation, ulcers and the digestive tract. Contain betacarotene, calcium, folic acid, magnesium, phosphorus, potassium, vitamins C and E.

WATERCRESS One of the best foods for purifying the blood. It has a high iodine content and the highest nutrient content of most greens. Good added to juices.

WILD RICE/BROWN RICE An excellent source of protein, especially for vegetarians. Full of B vitamins and fibre, it also contains iodine, potassium, selenium, tryptophan (an amino acid) and vitamin E. Brown rice's incredible absorption means it will soak up toxins in your gut.

WILD SALMON, TROUT, MACKEREL AND TUNA Their fatty acids protect against heart disease and strokes and are critical to brain and mood development and help create feelings of well-being.

YOGHURT AND PROBIOTIC DRINKS Promote the growth of 'good bacteria to boost immune systems and keep guts healthy'.

8

Foods models always avoid

It was in the early 1960s that the first convenience meals came into our lives. A powdered mulch, which morphed into an exotic 'curry' with the addition of hot water, pioneered the rocky road to pre-prepared food. Hot, tasteless and highly desired, it became the Versace of instant meals.

In the 1970s there were two technological breakthroughs that continued the rot. First, the Japanese exploited high-fructose corn syrup, which is six times sweeter than cane sugar and, because it was processed from corn, far cheaper to produce. Soon the giant American canned drinks manufacturers had switched their sweeteners to 100 per cent high-fructose corn syrup from a 50/50 blend of corn syrup and sugar, meaning they could save on costs, boost portion sizes and still make profits. Alas, this kind of fructose has the unforeseen quality of not breaking down in the digestive system and arriving almost intact in the liver.

The second technological breakthrough was the commercial development of a fat known as palm oil. Supermarkets particularly like products made with it as they're cheaper and have a much longer shelf life. Naturally, they're happy to overlook the fact that it's more highly saturated than pig fat and that it sends blood pressure spiralling and clogs up arteries.

On top of that came a huge increase in the size of food portions called 'large-sizing'. The food industry thinks bigness is addictive to us because they believe we think it represents power. Boosted by fast-food marketing men, the food industry pushed quantity not quality – more for less: jumbo portions and 'combo' meal deals. But enough is never enough. Penn State University found that if portion sizes were increased, people simply ate more. It revealed that consumption had little to do with hunger or how much people needed to eat but depended on how much was on their plates.

The microwave and the freedom to 'order in' have removed us from kitchen tyranny and have had a catastrophic effect on our diet and health. Forty per cent of the average American's food budget is spent on takeaways, and fat consumption has doubled in the last 20 years. Two thousand new snack products a year hit the market in a constant drip-feed of fat and sugar. Perversely, we love to watch glamorous television chefs show us how to cook, but it remains a voyeuristic pleasure. Conversely, the French and Italians have always been so successful in protecting their indigenous food cultures. Paris and Milan are important, essential workplaces on the international modelling circuit, and it is in these two cities that a supermodel inevitably and unavoidably begins her sensual, gradual, love affair with good food.

> *'I always cook when I'm at home and shop in markets and the local butcher rather than at supermarkets.'*
>
> *Jodie Kidd*

The French authorities keep alive their markets, small producers and specialist food retail shops by using special laws to safeguard them against the large supermarket chains, and in Italy they talk about food in much the same way as we talk about the weather: what they ate yesterday, what they'll eat tomorrow, and whether it will be as good as what they're eating today. These two gastronomically literate countries can teach us a lot. They instinctively know the difference between good and bad food. Italian cuisine is simple and uncomplicated, and, because of that, the prima quality of the ingredients is essential.

Living and working in France and Italy teaches models consciously to eat well, to take pleasure in something they do every day, and to stop treating food as a pit stop, as a refuelling to give them the energy for more important matters. *Food* is a more important matter.

How to shift your attitude to food

- Choose organic, fresh, seasonal food when you can. Fast food, fatty meat and fried foods are low in vital energy.

The foods with the most prana, or vital, energy are fresh fruit, vegetables, grains, nuts and seeds.

■ If you know you have bad food habits, such as overdosing on coffee or chocolate, don't try to give them all up at once. Instead of five cups of coffee, make it four, and gradually substitute your healthier options.

■ Eat with awareness. Don't gulp food down or eat on the run. Sit down and really take notice of your food with all your senses. How does it look, smell, feel and taste in your mouth?

■ Be grateful for the wide and wonderful choice of foods available to you every day, and take pleasure in choosing as diverse a selection of interesting taste sensations as possible. Try things you've never tried before – you'll be surprised.

■ Take time to prepare simple fresh food for yourself. Lots of takeaways and pre-prepared food will drain your vitality and add on the pounds.

■ Stay away from food that is soft, fluffy and white – sugar, white flour, white pasta, too much dairy – it will do the same for your body.

Say no to doctored dishes

The great new hope of the cunning international food corporations is 'functional foods'. Realising that we can't possibly eat any more than we are already, the food industry is always thinking of ingenious new ways to make us spend more money on the same amount of food. So now we have chocolate mousse with added vitamins, water with added calcium and low-fat spreads that claim to battle heart disease. Ironically, it's this dubious advance of technology that's contributing to the welcome rise in popularity of traceable, seasonal, artisan and organic foods, and a resurgence in the traditional breeds of livestock and poultry. At last, we're beginning to realise that no technology in the world can match the flavour and goodness of traditionally and humanely raised meat, and fresh, unadulterated food. The future lies in the battle against industrial farming and food processing. So put your palate before your purse.

Mass-produced white bread

The simple way to test the quality of your bread is to squish it between your fingers, and if it springs back then that's good bread – sadly, not the case with your standard sliced white. As well as the usual flour, water, salt and yeast, it contains a wealth of weird chemicals, preservatives and improvers. Not surprisingly, sliced white bread takes more nutrients to digest than it gives you, and provides the perfect environment for unfriendly bacteria in your stomach.

Vinegar is used to keep the bread fresh for longer; emulsifiers keep it soft, as well as improving crumb structure; food colouring, made from snail shells, gives it that scary white colour; flavour enhancers impart a 'freshly baked' smell; and other chemicals smooth out the flour and retard mould growth. These additives allow us to keep the bread longer (yeah, great – more of it tomorrow), make it look 'nice and uniform', and guarantee it tastes like used cotton wool.

Identify the additives

Around 90 per cent of additives in processed food are cosmetic, despite the food industry telling us that the use of additives is to protect consumers from food poisoning. In fact the additives used as preservatives or to stop fat going rancid amount to less than 1 per cent by weight of all the additives used. The vast majority are used to make cheap fat, constipating starch and subsidised sugars look and taste like natural food.

Every country must legally identify its additives on food labels and it's wise to avoid processed foods with chemical ingredients you don't recognise or understand. Watch out for contents that may include:

■ Artificial colourings

■ Preservatives

■ Bulkers, thickeners, emulsifiers and gelling agents

■ Flavour enhancers

■ Salts and related compounds

■ Surface coating agents, gases and sweeteners

MSG

We use to think the synthetic crystalline, monosodium glutamate (E621) was found only in Chinese foods and canned soups, but MSG has spread to many different foods under disguised names. Devoid of any nutritional or preservative value, food companies use MSG to flavour, hide unwelcome tastes and cover inferior ingredients used in products.

When you're eating out and seem to feel worse than when you eat at home, even though you order all the right foods, suspect MSG. It can actually alter your mood because it affects the nerve endings in the brain, causing headaches, nausea, diarrhoea, mood changes, flushing of the skin, memory loss and numbness. Ask your chemist for test strips to insert into your foods to see if MSG is present in its synthetic form.

The truth behind those food labels

'Better well-being', 'greater alertness', 'improves your memory', 'preserves youth', 'halves your calorie intake'… go on, admit it, you've fallen for it once or twice. If you really want to know what you're eating, read the product's small print and don't be taken in by any of these a moment longer:

BIO Usually found on pots of yoghurt but there are no rules about what this label actually means, or when it may be used. Yoghurt is live – it's a culture, so it's stating the obvious.

FARM-FRESH OR BARN-FRESH EGGS These terms have no legal meaning and the eggs may well have been laid by battery hens subject to overcrowding and routine de-beaking, and that have been kept indoors throughout their lives. Look for 'organic *and* free-range' eggs: they're laid by very content hens.

FRESH, PURE, NATURAL, FARMHOUSE, HOME-MADE
These are simply marketing terms not defined by law, and they can confuse and mislead. We don't expect items labelled 'fresh' to have a four-week shelf life or 'pure' to have added ingredients, or supermarkets with in-store bakeries to heat up frozen products made elsewhere and call them 'freshly baked'.

'HEALTHY' CEREAL LOGOS Many cereal packs carry claims that they're good for the heart, healthy bones, concentration, and so on. But they're 40 per cent sugar and the healthy bones claim is based on the fact that they're eaten with milk.

'HEALTHY' SNACKS Chocolate bad, muesli good, is the mantra we repeat to ourselves as we hand over our change for a cereal bar. However, muesli bars are often packed with sugar and additives and many of them contain more calories than well-known chocolate bars.

LIGHT OR LITE Can still be packed with fats and sugars. Will soon be banned outright if a product doesn't have at least 30 per cent less fat than the original version.

LOW FAT There is no law against a product being labelled 'low fat'. Food Standards Agency guidelines say it can be used with products that are less than 3g (1/16oz) of fat per 100g (4oz).

LOW SALT AND REDUCED SALT Should contain 25 per cent less salt than the regular version.

NO ADDED SUGAR Doesn't necessarily mean a low sugar content; often contains artificial sweeteners, such as aspartame.

REDUCED FAT No legal definition. If a product has had fat removed, it will often have had something added, such as sugar and thickening agents.

TRADITIONAL OR HERITAGE MEATS Has no legal meaning but may imply that the meat has been matured or hung for longer.

85 PER CENT FAT-FREE Sounds healthy but means the product is 15 per cent fat – a high level.

When bad means bad

It's mighty puzzling when diet books say there's no such thing as 'bad' and 'good' food. Can a sausage made of pig snout, eyeball, scrotum, and pink dye be good for you? Only if you've no other choice, I'd say.

That pert little cocktail sausage on a stick you daintily popped in your mouth at your last drinks party has a macabre history. It begins its life as raw, de-gristled pork, delivered to the factory in huge, shrink-wrapped plastic sacks, frozen solid. This is thawed and hacked into smaller pieces by a machine, and is the only part of the cocktail sausage that is recognisable as meat – it forms a mere 10 per cent of the finished product. The rest is animal leftovers, all manner of fat and MRM (mechanically recovered meat). A high-pressure water jet extracts this from every crevice of the carcass creating a liquid slurry to which is added chicken skins and bacon trimmings. Then 30 per cent of 'Continental pork fat' (fat trimmed from Danish ham) is added to the recipe, together with potato starch and dark red food colouring to give it its perky pink colour.

Real ice cream — fat chance

Oh, for a pure American ice cream, then. Well, they're not without their drawbacks either. Most of us know ice creams are fattening, but we're often seriously in the dark about the fat and calorie value of ice cream treats, because no labelling is required. We're all aware that ice cream is a treat, not a health food, but did you know that a mint chip 'Dazzler' from Häagen-Dazs has 1,270 calories and 38g (1½oz) of saturated fat – the equivalent of a T-bone steak, plus Caesar salad, baked potato and sour cream? Or that a Häagen-Dazs banana split with three scoops of ice cream, some syrup and two toppings – peanut and chocolate crunchies – is 1,100 calories – more than your entire daily allowance if you're on a 1,000 calories a day diet?

In the old days your 'soft whip' from the corner shop contained around 65 calories and 2g (⅒oz) of saturated fat.

Artificially sweet

Not all sugar substitutes have a sweet nature. Some are nasty pieces of work – downright unstable, sickly and unsafe – but one or two are born natural sweeties. Here's the low-down on what's behind the trade label:

ACESULFAME K Used with aspartame to sweeten diet fizzy drinks and diet foods. It's 130 times sweeter than sugar, but with hardly any calories. The little research conducted on its safety shows it can cause carcinogenic changes in animals.

Health factor: unknown, as not enough research carried out. Avoid.

Taste factor: sweet, lingering taste in mouth; no bitter aftertaste.

ASPARTAME 200 times sweeter than sugar. Used widely in products and marketed under trade names in America and Europe. In the body it releases aspartic acid, which acts as a neurotransmitter to stimulate nerves.

Health factor: researchers are concerned it may 'over-excite nerves', killing brain cells and nervous tissue. It can cause headaches, depression, fatigue and anxiety. Avoid.

Taste factor: sweet taste; no bitter aftertaste.

CYCLAMATE Used in soft drinks. Rats in lab tests developed testicular damage.

Health factor: use sparingly and well diluted or avoid altogether.

Taste factor: intense sweetness.

FRUISANA Sold in the form of white crystals and contains fructose – the form of sugar found naturally in fruit and honey. Provides a more sustained and constant supply of energy than sugar because it's natural and therefore enters the blood slowly preventing blood-sugar imbalances.

Health factor: a third sweeter than sugar, so you need less.

Taste factor: tastes like normal sugar; can be used in anything from tea and juices to baking cakes.

SACCHARIN Marketed under trade names in the Western world, is 300 times as strong as sugar, but with no calories. Truly artificial, it comes from petroleum. Is absorbed into the body, but excreted in the kidneys.

Health factor: proposed ban after studies suggested link with bladder tumours in rats, but saved by public demand, and latest research shows it to be safe.

Taste factor: strong intense sweetness and a slightly bitter aftertaste.

SUCRALOSE 600 times sweeter than sucrose, but its manufacturers claim it's not absorbed by the body so is non-calorific. However, the American Food and Drug Administration say 10–27 per cent may be absorbed, making it risky.

Health factor: few human safety studies; research on animals has shown abnormal cell growth. Avoid.

Taste factor: a lot like sugar, but more intense.

XYLITOL A natural sugar, extracted from the birch tree, which actively fights tooth decay by preventing bacteria from sticking to the teeth. Increasingly recognised as a wonder sweetener, it has 40 per cent fewer calories than table sugar, helps to stabilise blood sugar and lowers insulin. Xylitol has a low glycaemic index of seven (sugar has 100) and metabolises almost totally independently of insulin, which reduces bingeing and sweet cravings.

Health factor: hooray! The way to go. Get it from health stores or see my website.

Taste factor: slightly sharper sweetness than sugar. A great way to combine something sweet with cleaning your teeth.

Overhyped, overpriced and over here

The packaged low-carb invasion has hit us. From breakfast cereals to cakes, from biscuits to bread rolls, the supermarket shelves are now groaning with reduced-carbohydrate food for fans of high-protein diets. But watch out! If you take flour out of a bread, cake or biscuit recipe, you have to put something else in, which is usually protein, like soy. But surprise, surprise, the replacement protein has 4 calories per 100g (4oz), the same as the carbohydrate in the flour that was taken out. Although the label can state that, say, a bowl of reduced-carbohydrate breakfast cereal has 70 per cent less carbohydrate than a regular bowl, you still end up with the same number of calories as you find in a bowl of 'ordinary' sugar-coated breakfast cereal.

Ground nuts might be added to foods, such as bread rolls, to give extra bulk, which raises calories further as well as the protein. Sugar alcohols, such as maltitol or sorbitol, are also substituted. These are types of sugary carbohydrates that, makers argue, don't raise blood-sugar levels, and should therefore not count as carbohydrates at all.

That's why they subtract all sugar alcohols from the carbohydrate total to give a 'net effective carbs' figure, which is plastered all over the packaging. The Atkins Chocolate Chip Crisp Bar says '2g Net Carbs' on its pack. It actually supplies 22.5g (¾oz) of carbohydrate, but the net carb calculation only 'counts' the 2g that occur as sugar. It still supplies 137 calories, the same as eating a standard muesli bar.

The makers will argue that carbs, such as sugar alcohols and protein replacements, help to keep blood-sugar levels even, but you can do this by giving up cakes, sweets, biscuits and refined junk and having three healthy meals a day instead.

Don't overlook the overcooked

When you cook food to the point of browning or charring, the organic compounds it contains undergo changes in structure, producing carcinogens. You could be ingesting grams (ounces) of overcooked food that are far more dangerous than the half a gram of carcinogens inhaled by a smoker of two packs of cigarettes a day. Barbecued meat is the worst offender. When burning fat drips on to an open flame, dangerous carcinogens named PAHs are formed, and when amino acids and other chemicals found in muscle are exposed to high temperatures, other carcinogens called HAAs are created.

Barbecue tips

- Cook small pieces of meat. A chunk of chicken that's black on the outside but raw in the middle is a disaster waiting to happen.
- Use separate utensils to avoid contamination from raw meat to ready-to-eat food.
- Don't drizzle marinades over meat as it cooks. It contaminates the cooking meat with germs that could be still present in the marinade.

- Flip burgers frequently. It accelerates the cooking process and kills bacteria.
- Never eat burgers that are pink in the middle.
- Wash your hands after putting raw meat on the barbecue before making a salad.
- Never put cooked food back on the plate used for the raw meat.

How models avoid chemical calories

A lettuce is likely to contain many more chemicals than an avocado. Delicate lettuces are sprayed repeatedly with fattening pesticides and preservatives to keep them looking fresh on supermarket shelves. But thick-skinned avocados are much more robust and need little intervention, thus avoiding chemical calories. The solution is to go organic. Fruit and vegetables grown with few synthetic chemical sprays also contain more vitamins and tend to be higher in natural sugars making them sweeter, and more rewarding than their intensively grown counterparts.

'I avoid foods labelled 'low fat' because I think that small amounts of full-fat butter, cream and cheese are much more beneficial and taste better. They register more swiftly with the taste buds and hypothalamus (the hunger-control centre in the brain) meaning you feel fuller faster.'

Catherine Hurley

Keep your intake of animal fats low, especially if non-organic, and try to buy less intensively farmed produce. Environmental pollutants accumulate in animals and tend to be stored in fatty tissue. Many organochlorines are highly fat-soluble so more pesticides are likely to lurk in fatty meat. Grilling rather than frying meat helps to get rid of the fat and some chemicals.

> **TIP** Always use glass, stainless steel, or iron pans when preparing food in the kitchen, and never use aluminium cookware or utensils. Food cooked or stored in aluminium produces a substance that neutralises digestive juices, leading to acidosis and ulcers.
>
> Aluminium can leach from the container into the food and then be absorbed by the body, and accumulate in the brain and nervous-system tissues. Excessive amounts of these aluminium deposits have been implicated in causing Alzheimer's disease.

Most food is now sold in plastic boxes or covered in plastic because it's cheap, weighs little, is hardwearing and waterproof. During the manufacturing process, chemicals are added to make the plastic soft, flexible and fire retardant. If this packaging is stored for a long time or exposed to high temperatures, chemicals from the plastic can leach into food.

Remove plastic packaging as soon as you can and store food in ceramic or glass containers. Chemicals can leach into food from plastic containers and so can the ink printed on plastic. Don't drink hot liquids from polystyrene or plastic cups and avoid using small plastic portions of milk or cream with tea and coffee. Heat makes the chemicals in plastic or polystyrene leach into the drink.

Also steer clear of fish oils in supplements unless you're sure the chemical content has been removed. Good brands don't contain farmed fish oils but fresh, deep-water fish that have been frozen at $-50^{o}C$ to remove impurities.

Foods that clash

It's a common misconception that models drastically diet before they take to the catwalks to show the new designer collections each season. On the contrary, they eat more nourishing food than ever to keep up their energy levels. If you've ever experienced the back-stage scramble of changing an entire outfit and hair in just eight seconds, and doing this at least ten times in one show, or been photographed for six hours in the snowy Scottish highlands wearing nothing but a wispy chiffon evening dress, you'll know it can't be done on an empty stomach.

What models do watch out for are foods that don't work well together, that can cause bloating and discomfort when combined, or that deplete or cancel out their mutual vitamin and mineral benefits, minimising energy levels. Here are some of them:

CHEESE AND GREEN VEGETABLES Broccoli, courgettes (zucchini) and most green vegetables are rich sources of calcium and magnesium, but the calcium in cheese is difficult for the body to absorb. The high levels of fat and protein in the cheese can inhibit the uptake of the calcium in the vegetables. Go for vegetables covered in light cheese sauces, such as cauliflower cheese, and avoid combinations that contain equal amounts of vegetables and cheese, such as some pizzas.

ALCOHOL AND SHELLFISH Oysters, in particular, are rich sources of zinc, important for immunity and hormone balance. But if you drink champagne with oysters, the health benefits are almost wiped out by the alcohol. Zinc can't be absorbed if you've consumed alcohol. Other zinc foods include Brazil nuts, egg yolk, peanuts and oats. Eating these with spinach also prevents zinc absorption.

FIZZY DRINKS AND FRUIT AND NUT SNACKS Nuts, seeds and raisins are rich sources of iron, which enables red blood cells to carry oxygen around the body. But don't wash them down with fizzy drinks. These contain high levels of phosphates that bind to iron in the gut, preventing absorption.

CEREAL AND COFFEE Seeds, nuts and whole grains are among our best sources of B vitamins, zinc, iron and folic acid. But tannins in tea and coffee bind to these nutrients, so they can't be absorbed when taken together. A strong cup of either, before breakfast, can reduce nutrient absorption by more than half. Whenever you can, wait at least 40 minutes after breakfast before you have your first cuppa.

MEAT AND SOFT FRUIT Melons, mangoes, grapes and other soft fruits will ferment if you put them in a warm, acidic environment, like the stomach. Meat dramatically raises stomach acidity, so if it's eaten within 30 minutes of soft fruit then the fruit will begin to ferment, causing bloating and discomfort. It's better to eat soft fruit either 30 minutes before a meal or more than two hours after.

Part Three
Shaped for Life

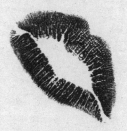

'When you are younger you do what you need to
do to look good, but as you get older and wiser
you do what you need to do to live a long time.'

Elle Macpherson
From supermodel to superbusiness woman

Part Three
Shaped for Love

9

How to shop, stock and flop

You know that feeling – you crawl home from work completely knackered, and you're ravenous. The fridge is empty apart from some half-eaten lasagne, so you open your cupboards and come across cans, not just past their sell-by date but so old and sticky they're bonded to the woodwork. And you vow, yet again, to do The Big Spring Clean and stock up 'sensibly'.

Now imagine you're a hungry supermodel, arriving at your flat at midnight in Paris, because you've just flown in from your apartment in New York, and after working tomorrow you're taking off for your base in Milan, which you haven't visited for a month, and then on to your flat in London, via a location job in Tuscany. Sounds great? No way, it's lonely and exhausting. Unlike their iconic Hollywood sisters, supermodels don't have personal chefs to travel with them, assistants to organise their shopping, live-in nutritionists monitoring their every mouthful, or lifestyle coaches doing whatever they do. What they do have are invaluable tricks for stocking and shopping so they'll always have nourishing food available at home, wherever home may be, even if they haven't been there for a month. Their clever strategies ensure they're never caught out, ending up eating rubbish because they're starving hungry.

> *'I live on a Caribbean island, and if the boat doesn't come in with provisions, there are groceries we won't get, so stocking up sensibly is of major importance in my life.'*
>
> **India Hicks**

It probably sounds odd to stock up with more, when you're probably trying to eat less, but a bare cupboard spells trouble – there's always a bag of crisps lurking around or that chocolate in your bag to scoff instead. The trick to it all is to have the right selection of essentials on hand so that you can throw together a simple, tasty meal without having to rush to the corner shop for dodgy provisions.

Fast food doesn't have to mean junk food, and convenience doesn't have to come in ready-to-microwave packs or boilable plastic bags. Even if you're not a great cook, like the supermodel Amber Valetta, a bit of imagination, a well-stocked store cupboard and a freezer are all you need to produce good meals in minutes.

The big cull

It's no good stocking up before you've cleaned out the old stuff. Think of your kitchen cupboards in the same way as you view your wardrobe. If you haven't used it for ages, you won't miss it and you don't need it.

Cans are easy; if they're past their sell-by date, bin them. Dried pasta and rice will last up to a year and unopened olive oils also have a good two years' life if kept away from sunlight. White flour should be chucked out and replaced with cornflour or soya flour (less fattening and better for you), which should then be stored in an airtight glass jar. Bin all those silly bottles of dipping sauces and assorted barbecue marinades that have begun to smell fishy through lack of use, and keep all jars you've already opened – from mustards to jams – in the fridge. This lets you know they're there to be used up before they lose their flavour, and stops them festering at the back of your cupboards.

Be ruthless with spices and herbs; if they're not stored in airtight containers they end up with all the flavour of sawdust. Do the sniff test, if it smells of nothing it's useless.

The way to keep herbs, if you can't keep them growing on your kitchen window ledge, is to buy them fresh, freeze them and use when needed. Store spices in their original forms and grind them as you go, because once they're ground they quickly lose their flavour. Buy a garlic plait and hang it in the kitchen – it lasts for months and makes it look like you can cook.

Can-do

•••

If opening a can doesn't sound like the sort of thing a supermodel would do and you immediately associate can openers with spaghetti hoops or canned mince the cat would love, you're missing something.

Some food in cans is really amazing. There are luxury foods that have been preserved this way since canning was invented in 1810 by Frenchman Nicholas Appert of L'Art de Conserver. The Spanish are brilliant at canning. Their cans of sea urchins are sublime, and much of the Spanish food in cans, especially anchovies, tuna and sardines, tastes as good as fresh; some foods actually benefit from the canning process. Here are the best buys for your store cupboard:

CARROTS Although great eaten raw, steamed and roasted, carrots are actually at their healthiest canned. Canning softens the carrots' tough cell walls, making their orange pigment, an antioxidant called betacarotene, easier to digest.

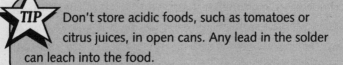

TIP Don't store acidic foods, such as tomatoes or citrus juices, in open cans. Any lead in the solder can leach into the food.

BEANS The most useful addition to your store cupboard. Don't always think baked, think red kidney beans – they're enormously versatile, rich in all nutrients, protein and the richest in fibre of all beans. Also try cannellini, borlotti, black-eyed, and flageolet. Chickpeas are great because they're rich in supernutrients called saponins.

Canned beans are more user-friendly and safer than dried beans, because processing completely destroys a toxin that can cause sickness if the dried beans aren't boiled enough. Try to find cans with reduced salt and sugar, and always rinse the beans in cold water before use.

FISH Healthiest canned in spring water or tomato sauce. A good source of vitamin B_{12}. Most canned oily fish has more vitamin D than fresh, because the canning makes the small, vitamin D-rich bones in fish edible as they dissolve into the flesh. It also retains much of its omega-3 essential oils. Canned salmon is lower in fat and saturated fat than fresh, steamed salmon, has 50 per cent more iodine, 75 per cent more calcium and 50 per cent more vitamin A, but it's higher in salt than fresh.

FRUIT Canned prunes are a good source of iron and folic acid, and grapefruit, mandarins and pineapple retain more vitamin C when canned because of their acidic nature. Whole canned apricots contain twice as much vitamin C, weight for weight, as fresh apricots and almost twice as much calcium. Never buy canned fruit in syrup but preserved in its own juice with no added sugar.

PULSE-BASED SOUPS, such as split pea and lentil, are low in fat, and, when eaten with a starchy carbohydrate, such as crackers or matzos, provide a good source of protein. Also, the soluble fibre creates a satisfying feeling of fullness.

Sweetcorn often tastes better from the can than the fresh stuff. It's versatile and sweet even without added sugar and salt.

TOMATOES Healthiest canned. Tomatoes are rich in a supernutrient called lycopene, which also becomes easier to digest after the canning process. Lycopene has anti-ageing properties – it's stored in the skin and reflects some of the sun's harmful and ageing ultraviolet rays.

> **TIP** Dear old friend though it is, Heinz canned tomato soup contains three teaspoons of sugar per serving and a huge amount – 9.4g (¼oz) – of fat. Love it from afar, and allow Andy Warhol, not your stomach, to preserve your fond memories of a tomato soup can.

When frozen beats fresh

If you don't have a fair-sized freezing compartment incorporated in your fridge, change it. The money you'll save by stocking the freezer sensibly will pay for its cost in no time, and the food you'll keep in it is often as good as, and in many cases better than, its fresh or manufactured counterpart.

Frozen fruit and vegetables with their 'goodness preserved' can be healthier than unseasonal fresh ones flown in from abroad. Better value for money, they're generally less contaminated by pesticides, chemical fertilisers and heavy metals. Frozen peas contain more vitamin C than fresh, as do frozen green beans. Blast freezing at very cold temperatures for a short time is also very successful with broccoli, cauliflower, sweetcorn and raspberries, but not with other soft fruit, cabbage or carrots.

A recent test revealed that the vitamin content of frozen peas, cauliflower, beans, sweetcorn and carrots was substantially higher than that of fresh imports from several overseas countries. Fresh vegetables lose nutrients such as vitamin C every day that they're travelling from faraway places.

Bread, cheese, nuts and seeds

A favourite trick of models is to keep their bread in the freezer. That way they can only eat what they thaw out. Bread freezes well and, even after long spells away from home, the girls know they can have some wholemeal toast within a few minutes of walking into their kitchen (you can toast from frozen). Parmesan, that superbly versatile cheese, also freezes beautifully and can be grated straight from the freezer. Nuts and seeds are nutritionally packed powerhouses, which stay fresher longer when you keep them in the freezer. Delicious, high in protein and healthy fats, they make brilliant snacks and dessert toppings, and are good in salads.

ALMONDS are the most nutritious of all nuts. They are high in potassium, magnesium, phosphorus and protein, and contain huge amounts of laetrile, an anti-cancer agent.

BRAZIL NUTS are rich in selenium with just three or four a day providing the recommended daily intake for women.

In 2004 they were banned by the European Union for having aflatoxin in their shells, which is considered carcinogenic. But who munches the shells?

CASHEW NUTS are packed with iron and zinc, essential for a robust immune system, fertility and good quality skin. They're high in magnesium, vitamin A and, er, fat. Be discerning.

CHESTNUTS are unique in the nut world because of their low fat content. Nearly 90 per cent of their calories come from carbohydrates, making them a good choice for refuelling after a physical workout or as part of a low-fat diet.

HAZELNUTS are extremely rich in calcium and vitamin E, which helps to protect cell walls from free-radical damage caused by stress, pollution and too much sun.

> **TIP** Try to buy nuts with their shells still on. Opening them takes time, so you're less likely to scoff the lot in one go.

LINSEEDS are so beneficial, most models eat them every day. Their high absorption capacity provides the body with bulk, which helps maintain digestive regularity, and the mucins provide a protective layer for the intestines.

Sitting for hours on planes with no possibility of exercise, and mediocre food presented at regular intervals, plays havoc with a model's digestive system, and a heaped dessertspoonful of organic linseeds on cereal, yoghurt, soup or salad each day keeps the system healthy the natural way.

PEANUTS are a complete protein, but have the highest fat content of all nuts, apart from the macadamia nut, so not the best choice.

PINE NUTS are chewy and sweet, making them good for salads or combined with fruits.

WALNUTS protect your skin because they contain the mineral copper, needed to make melanin, the skin pigment that helps protect against harmful UV radiation.

More good freezers

Chicken breasts, salmon steaks, cooked prawns and crab meat (the real thing) also keep well in the freezer, and can be pre-portioned, so you can defrost the correct amount for a meal. Game birds, such as pheasants, freeze brilliantly, which is just as well, as the season when you can buy them fresh is very short. Fresh herbs, such as basil, coriander (cilantro), chives, and flat-leaf parsley (more flavourful than curly parsley), can be frozen too.

Stock up on frozen, unsweetened berries and use them just before they've completely thawed. Different types of fruit can be frozen to eat as a snack. Cut whole fruit into bite-sized pieces and place on a baking tray in the freezer until firm, then put them in resealable freezer bags. Sliced pineapple is extremely good, also extra-large seedless grapes, melons, peaches, plums and mangoes (but nothing citrus). Bananas are brilliant and are great thickeners. Eat them straight from the freezer or purée them into a slush to make a smoothie.

Freezer damage limitation

You've had a hard week, you're tired, grumpy and need cheering up, and you've simply got to have chocolate – lots of it. Before you do something drastic, try this. It's the ultimate answer for curbing your sweet cravings, because the volume of the drink stretches your stomach, sending messages to your brain that you're full.

*1 sachet low-fat chocolate instant drinking powder
ice cubes
half a frozen banana, cut into chunks
250ml (8fl oz) soya or semi-skimmed milk*

*METHOD
Dissolve the chocolate sachet in a little hot water in a cup then fill halfway with cold water. Pour into a blender or food processor, add some ice cubes, the frozen banana chunks and milk. Blend for about 60 seconds. Pour into a glass and drink.*

Told you so.

Storecupboard meals
•••

These are meals you can make with your eyes closed, straight from your kitchen cupboard. They're typical of the meals models throw together, good emergency stand-bys when the alternatives are chemical 'ready meals' or fillers, such as crisps and chocolate. Your friends won't be gagging for the recipes but they're nourishing, filling, quick and pure.

Chickpea and pasta stew
Serves two

150g (5oz) of small pasta shapes such as conchiglie (shells) or farfalle (bowties) or penne (hollow tubes)

2 × 400g (14oz) cans chopped tomatoes

400g (14oz) can chickpeas or other beans, drained and rinsed

300g (11oz) frozen mixed vegetables

2.5ml (½ tsp) each of dried oregano and dried basil

550ml (18fl oz) boiling water, plus more as needed

METHOD

1   Throw all the ingredients in a medium-sized pan. Place over a medium heat and bring to the boil.

2   Reduce the heat to low and simmer for 20–30 minutes, stirring occasionally, until the pasta is just cooked. Add more water during cooking if it begins to dry out.

Spaghetti with anchovy and tuna

Serves four

350g (12oz) spaghetti

30ml (2 tbsp) olive oil

2 garlic cloves, cut into quarters

4 anchovy fillets, drained if in oil

250g (9oz) canned tuna in olive oil, drained

50ml (2fl oz) white wine

50g (2oz) capers, rinsed and drained

2 tomatoes, diced or 1 small can of chopped tomatoes

10 basil leaves (frozen is fine)

30ml (2 tbsp) extra virgin olive oil

sea salt and freshly ground black pepper

METHOD

1   Cook the spaghetti in a large pan of boiling salted water
    until *al dente* (about 8 minutes). Meanwhile, heat the olive
    oil in a frying pan, add the garlic and fry over a gentle heat
    for 3 minutes.

2   Add the anchovies and cook until almost melting. Increase
    the heat and add the tuna. Toss for a few minutes, then
    add the wine and let it bubble to allow the alcohol to
    evaporate. Stir in the capers and tomatoes.

3   Drain the pasta, reserving 30–45ml (2–3 tbsp) of the
    water. Toss the pasta with the sauce, mix in the basil and
    extra virgin olive oil, and season. Add the water to
    moisten, if necessary.

TIP

■ Avoid pasty pasta by cooking it in a large pan of rapidly boiling water and when it's just cooked (*al dente*) run the pasta under hot, not cold water before draining, to prevent stickiness. Try whole-wheat pastas – they're better than you think.

■ When a recipe calls for rice, remember you have a choice of short or long grain. The short is best in recipes that need to hold together, such as risotto, because it's stickier, whereas long grain stays separate, so is suitable as an accompaniment. In salads either short or long grain is delicious.

Quick bean salad

Serves two

1 small can of red kidney beans, flageolets, chickpeas and sweetcorn, drained

30–45 ml (2–3 tbsp) good quality mint sauce (low sugar, shop-bought is fine)

METHOD

1 Chuck the contents of the cans of beans in a colander and rinse with water. Drain, put in a bowl and add the mint sauce.

2 A chopped fresh red (bell) pepper and sliced spring onions (scallions) can also be added for some extra crunch.

Garlic bread

Serve garlic bread to accompany any of the meals above.

Serves two
2 palm-sized slices of ciabatta or French bread
2 garlic cloves, crushed
10ml (2 tsp) olive oil
10ml (2 tsp) freshly grated Parmesan cheese

METHOD

1   Defrost the ciabatta or French bread.
    Preheat the grill (broiler) and mix together the garlic cloves
    and olive oil.

2   Spread one-quarter of the mixture on to both sides of each
    slice of bread. Top each slice with 5ml (1 tsp) grated
    Parmesan cheese. Grill (broil) for about 1 minute or until
    the topping goes brown.

Quick fish toasts

I love the idea of serving good quality fish, such as
anchovies, mackerel and tuna, straight from the can.
Simply toast some defrosted bread, preferably sour dough,
such as Poilane, spread on some lightly salted butter and
place the fish on top.

Or take a 50g (2oz) can of sardines, drained of any olive
oil, and place in a small bowl with a squeeze of lemon juice
and a few capers or sliced cornichons (baby gherkins).
Mash with a fork, season to taste with salt and pepper, and
spread the mixture on to some lightly buttered toast (buy

the soft butters, they go further). Served with a dark green salad containing bitter leaves, such as watercress, and some slices of avocado, this makes a great lunch any time.

Ready meals

It's convenient to buy chilled and frozen ready meals, and the variety gets more sophisticated by the minute. But very few deliver their promise. They never look like they do on the pack when you dish them up, and there's always that problem with quantities: one portion is never enough; two is too gross.

Most ready meals, including the 'healthy' type of ranges, are usually high in salt, and 'fat-free' doesn't mean low in calories. Extra sugars, refined carbohydrates and thickeners are often added to boost the flavour and texture, so calorie content may be only slightly less than, or similar to, that of standard products. A claim that food is 85 per cent fat-free means that it still contains 15 per cent fat – so it's not low-cal at all.

The answer is to make your own. 'I haven't got the time and she's got a deli, so she must love cooking,' I hear you mutter. Well I don't. I love squeezing, buying, selling, talking and eating food but I enjoy cooking about as much as I enjoy exercise – which is not a lot. But what I'm going to suggest is so easy, you can't not do it. All you need is to put aside one day a month, find yourself a large casserole or pan, and get a stack of 'one person' foil takeaway containers from your local supermarket.

When I was on the permanent treadmill of the international modelling circuit for ten years and working between Paris, New York, Milan and London, I used to 'one-pot' once a month at my home in each city and I can honestly say that it changed my life. It gives complete freedom from the hassle of regular shopping.

> *The best home comfort is curling up on a big comfy couch, chilling out in comfy tracksuit bottoms and eating good, hearty British food, like homemade shepherd's pie.'*
>
> *Elizabeth Jagger*

The beauty of the one-pot meal is that all the vitamins and minerals are retained in the sauce, and they're a doddle to make. They contain no additives whatsoever, and quick-frozen food loses none of its nutrients through the freezing process. You'll also save a fortune – the supermarket versions, quid pro quo, are outrageously expensive.

Think of your favourite one-pot meals that are filling without being fattening. I don't know what you like, but it could be, say, Spring Lamb Stew with baby carrots, small new potatoes, green beans, peas, tomatoes and fresh herbs. Or maybe a vegetarian Black-eyed Bean and Squash Stew or Red Thai Chicken Curry with Sweet Peppers and Bamboo Shoots, or a Spicy Mexican Chilli.

The trick is to make meals with not much peeling and chopping involved (a food processor helps chop large quantities of onions and other ingredients quickly), so you can throw it all into the casserole or pan and walk away while it cooks. One cooking session, making four different dishes, each with recipes for eight people (most recipes are for four, so just double everything), will give you enough meals for a month to freeze.

When the cooked contents of the casserole are cooled, decant them into the foil takeaway containers, scribble the initials of what's inside on the lid and freeze them. Then simply choose from one of your own 'prepared' meals whenever you're at home. Heat up the container, uncovered, in the oven preheated to 180°C/350°F/Gas 4, for 45 minutes, and enjoy a complete meal with no fuss, no additives, and no washing-up.

You can keep tabs on precisely what you're eating and you can knock up a salad or an additional vegetable while the pot meal is reheating. We sell heaps of these meals every week at my deli. See my website for recipe suggestions.

TIP Set aside one room and one chair for eating at home, even for a snack. If you eat in every room of the house, you create associations with food everywhere you go and set up the perfect opportunities to binge.

Kitchen essentials

If someone buys you another useless kitchen gadget, don't say 'Thanks', ask 'Why?' Our kitchens are littered with catalogue-bought nonentities to 'make life easier'.

Remember the electric carving knife? What's the betting the inventor isn't rushing to renew his annual international patents. The few items it makes sense to have around in your kitchen include:

- Sprays for each of your oils.

- A steamer for vegetables and fish.

- A blender for whipping up yoghurt and fruit desserts and smoothies.

- Small kitchen scales to get an idea of what portions look like.

'Ping' pongs

Your kitchen shelves are laden with cookbooks, but you still pick it up, drag it home, shove it in the microwave and, ping! dinner is served. But what's the real price for convenience? Recent tests showed that *microwaving* vegetables robs them of almost all their goodness. With broccoli it removes 97 per cent of its flavonoids, linked to reducing the risk of cancer, which seems ridiculous when steaming it would take only a few minutes longer. So what about other cooking methods?

BAKING is good for fish as long as the oven isn't too hot. High temperatures alter the biochemical structure of the essential fats in the fish, so cook it at a lower temperature, but for longer. Baking is also a good way to cook potatoes because we usually eat the skin, which is rich in fibre and helps to keep in their vitamin C content.

BOILING When boiling vegetables you need to cut them into larger pieces, as it reduces the surface area through which water-soluble vitamins, such as B and C, can leach out. Boil them for as short a time as possible, and don't keep them hot for hours, as prolonged heating destroys folates, which prevent heart disease.

FRYING is bad news, apart from the fatty food that obviously results. When you heat oils to high temperatures their chemical structure becomes deformed. It was once believed that olive oil did not deform in the same way as unsaturated fats, such as sesame seed oil or sunflower oil; but, it does, and this encourages free-radical damage in the body and can cause premature ageing.

ROASTING This is a simple and effective way to cook meat and vegetables, such as (bell) peppers, onions and aubergines (eggplant). But you must be careful not to burn the food, as anything burned is carcinogenic. Burned particles of food give rise to free radicals in the body, more than matched by the amount of antioxidants contained in the vegetables.

STEAMING is the preferred way to cook vegetables, because fewer nutrients are lost in the process and the vegetables retain their fibre, which is crucial for clearing excess toxins and cholesterol from the body and for keeping your bowels moving.

TIP
- Even when you've cooked chicken for the correct amount of time, there's often dark red colouring next to the bones. This bloody patch is due to pigments in the blood being released from the bones as it cooks. It's more common in meat that's been frozen and in younger birds whose bones are more porous.
- To check that roasted poultry is completely cooked, pierce the thickest part of the leg with a skewer or sharp knife; the juices should run clear. For chicken breasts pierce the thickest part of the breast to check the juices run clear.

How to be a better cook than you think you are

Don't you hate those cookery books brought out by highly trained chefs with 'easy recipes' which aren't? You know the kind of thing: preparation 56 minutes, cooking two hours, with lots of stirring, stuffing, chopping, peeling and adding things nobody outside a catering school has ever heard of. It's enough to put you off cooking for life.

A regular meal can be a very simple dish. It doesn't require tedious preparation or intricate presentation. When an aspiring young model came into my shop last week, I noticed she looked a trifle frantic. She'd recently been buying a large quantity of the frozen one-pot meals from us, and she came clean and told me she'd been reheating them for her new boyfriend, but pretending she'd made them herself. The new bloke was very impressed by her versatility, and the relationship was going well. Except that this particular evening he was coming round, in half an hour, to watch her cook. Making a cup of tea was the extent of her repertoire. I sliced her 100g (4oz) of top quality chorizo (spicy, Spanish sausage), gave her a 400g (14oz) can of chopped tomatoes, the same size can of chickpeas, an onion, a garlic clove, a handful of parsley and scribbled down the following:

Idiot-proof meal for a boyfriend

Chop and fry the onion. Chop and add the garlic. Chop and add the chorizo. Sizzle for a bit. Open the can of tomatoes and pour them into the pan, followed by the chickpeas. Chop and add parsley and cook for 5 minutes. Serve with Rioja, crusty bread and salad. Boyfriend stays the night.

- Don't let chopped garlic go brown when you cook it, or it will taste bitter.
- Never put onions and garlic in the pan at the same time, or the garlic will burn.
- To get rid of smelly onion/garlic hands, rub them with lemon wedges, parsley or salt, and then wash them in hot, soapy water.

You can't go wrong with the basic technique of frying onions and meat first, then adding flavour and, finally, topping up with liquid. It's quick, simple and has infinite adaptations. Go Greek with garlic, rosemary, lemon juice and yoghurt, or add the flavour of France with garlic, mustard and white wine, and then finish with some crème fraîche. Chicken with paprika, white wine and crème fraîche works well. Serve these meals with rice or pasta to save time scrubbing potatoes.

> **TIP**
> - Chicken pieces will be juicier if you use tongs to turn them during cooking. Using a fork will pierce them and allow the juices to run out.
> - Boning turkey and chicken is much easier with scissors than with a knife.
> - Skinless turkey contains about a third less fat than skinless chicken.

Good quality Indian and Thai curry pastes are brilliant for meals in minutes. Stir-fry sliced onions, strips of chicken, lean lamb or beef, add the curry paste and cover with water. With Thai dishes, instead of water, use a creamed coconut block rather than coconut milk, so you can add more water when you thin it. Throw in green beans and (bell) peppers.

The supermodels' favourite way of stir-frying is to use water with an added stock cube which guarantees a clean, delicious flavour. Top models also add lots of chopped ginger and garlic; both sensationally cleansing.

Chicken with mange tout (snow peas)

Serves four

For the marinade:

4 cloves of garlic (finely chopped)

2.5cm (1 inch) fresh ginger (finely chopped)

30ml (2 tbsp) low-salt soy sauce

45ml (3 tbsp) tablespoons dry sherry

180ml (12 tbsp) chicken stock (from 1½ good quality
   chicken stock cubes)

Freshly ground black pepper

4 medium chicken breasts (cut into thin strips)

150g trimmed mange tout (snow peas)

45ml (3 tbsp) dry sherry

10ml (2 tsp) cornflour

1 Mix the ingredients for the marinade, using only half the
   stock season with ground black pepper and place the
   chicken in the marinade for 15 minutes.

2 Meanwhile blanche the mange tout for one minute and
   drain.

3 Drain the marinade from the chicken and pour into a
   heated frying pan or wok and bring to the boil.

4 Add the chicken and stir-fry for three minutes, then add
   the mange tout.

5 Finally add the remaining half of the stock, dry sherry and
   cornflour and stir for 2 minutes or until the sauce thickens
   and serve at once with brown or basmati rice.

Twenty, fresh, uncooked tiger prawns, shelled and de-veined, also work well cooked this way with mange tout.

Marinating is a way of turning a quick-grilled steak or chops into something more special. Before leaving for work in the morning, put some chicken or lamb in a mix of lemon juice, olive oil, white wine, garlic, bay leaf, a sprig of rosemary, salt and pepper. It will be packed with flavour, naturally tenderised and ready to cook by the time you get home. If you accidentally overcook the meat, marinating it reduces the amount of carcinogens by up to 90 per cent, because the acids in the marinade protect the meat.

Good home habits

- Don't eat as much as you can; eat as much as you need.
- Don't finish something on your plate just because it's there.
- Keep all the food in the kitchen.
- Whatever you find most difficult to resist – crisps, chocolate, fizzy drinks – keep out of the house.

Smart shopping

Good butchers, greengrocers and fishmongers are becoming rare, as the supermarkets trample all in their path, but they're worth seeking out for their expertise, enthusiasm and judgement. Source produce from as near to your doorstep as possible. Support your local markets and farmers' markets if you don't want to digest a cocktail of chemicals found in intensively farmed foods. Food shopping should be fun and fascinating, not just a trudge down strip-lit aisles. Take pride in the produce of your country, preserve your culinary heritage!

When you shop at a supermarket, remember these few rules:

1. Always make a list and stick to it.

2. Avoid aisles where junk and processed food lurk.

3. Never go shopping when you're hungry.

4. Read the nutrition labels.

5. Be aware that 'low fat' usually means 'high carb'.

6. Avoid sweet or high-fat treats.

7. Never buy mega-sized or multi-packs.

The basic shopping list

Make yourself a basic list, stick it up on a wall in the kitchen, and then check against it each time you make a new list. It should read something like this:

balsamic vinegar	brown/wild rice
beans, canned red kidney	capers
beans, other canned	cereals
black peppercorns	chestnut purée
bread, organic wholegrain	chicken breasts

chilli sauce

cold-pressed olive oil

corn or soya flour

crispbread or oatcakes

dried fruits

fish, fresh/canned

fruit, including berries

garlic

ginger

herbs

hummus

linseeds

low-fat cocoa powder

low-fat coconut cream

low-salt bouillon powder

low-salt/fat soups

Manuka honey

mayonnaise

mineral water

muesli, unsweetened natural

mustard

noodles

nuts

organic and free-range eggs

pasta

pasta sauce

prawns, peeled

pure fruit juice

reduced-sugar ketchup

slightly salted butter

soy or tamari sauce

soya milk

spices

sugar substitute

sugar-free jam

sunflower oil

sweetcorn, canned

tea/green tea

tomato purée

vegetables, roots and greens

wine vinegar, red and white

Worcestershire sauce

yoghurt

10

Out and about

Let's face it, it's a hell of a lot easier to control the foods you eat in your own home, than what's 'out there' in the toxic environment. A healthy diet is not only about what, when and why you eat the foods you do, but also where you do it, and how you avoid temptation.

Models on the move have far more temptations to eat poor quality food than they do at home. In the world of studios, isolated locations, airports, planes, pit stops at cafés and kiosks, different time zones, different food choices, different food cultures and languages, and being just plain tired, it can sometimes be tough to stick to three healthy meals a day. It's not surprising, then, to learn that every supermodel realises the most important meal of the day is the first one. She knows that starting with a balanced breakfast controls her appetite and eating habits for the rest of the day, because it feeds her brain with nutrients that direct her body towards healthy foods.

'A model needs to kick-start her system before she rushes out to work, and does go-sees and fittings in her daily, busy life. Not eating breakfast can make her hypoglycaemic and sluggish. It's the most vital meal of the day.'

Sarah Doukas
Storm Model Agent

Until recently scientists assumed that missing breakfast was just a marker of a hectic life, or a way to try to lose weight, but the results of a recent study found that those who ate a proper breakfast regularly were significantly less likely to be obese, while those starting the day without food tended to smoke more, drink more alcohol and take less exercise.

When you eat breakfast, your body receives a clear message that it can get energy, and the metabolism is set for the day. The correct breakfast activates your metabolism to burn the calories you eat and produce the brain chemicals you need. The idea is to burn all the calories you eat so that your body doesn't store extra ones as fat.

The perfect breakfast

What models eat in the morning is as diverse as what they wear, but the one thing their breakfasts have in common is a combination of complex carbs, protein and fibre – because they know this mix will get them through until lunchtime without needing to snack. They choose slow-glycaemic foods, which provide slow-release energy, such as wholemeal (whole-wheat) bread, berries and almonds, and they go for 'complex carbs', such as wholegrain cereals that haven't been processed and take longer to digest.

TIP Always choose multigrain or granary bread because it contains whole grains of wheat with the fibrous husk intact. It takes much longer for the digestive enzymes to break through the husk and get to the starchy interior of the grain, and therefore allows a much slower rise in blood sugar.

The alternative to sugar-loaded muesli used to be those worthy, no-added-sugar-or-salt ones that taste like wood shavings and scour your innards clean as they go down. Luckily, they've improved no end, and small companies producing delicious cereals with added fruit from their own crops are more widely distributed to supermarkets, rather than simply supplying obscure health-food stores.

With breakfast, the trick is to make sure you combine your complex carbs with protein from eggs, milk or yoghurt, and with the fibre from fruit to maximise slowing your digestion and prolonging energy release. Don't skimp on any part of the trio or think you can get away with a muffin and an expresso. A muffin is pure carbohydrate, which means it's broken down too quickly and, once in your digestive system, turns to sugar, which will send your blood sugar soaring.

> *'My favourite breakfast is hot water with ginger or mint, followed by porridge with flaxseed (linseed) oil and wheatgerm. Then fruit and some toast made with German bread (which I bring back from jobs there), which has lots of crunchy nuts and seeds in it, with butter and honey. And a cup of tea.'*
>
> Catherine Hurley

An hour later your blood-sugar level will drop, leaving you reaching for mid-morning snacks. Choose a cappuccino or latte with skimmed milk first up because of the protein in the milk. If you eat carbohydrate on its own, or just go for a portion of protein or fibre, you won't have enough energy for the morning, and you certainly won't get through until lunchtime without a snack.

Snacks

'Snack' is one of those words that is a spot-on description of what it represents – a useless, tasteless, cheap little word, like snitch or snatch. You can, of course, make 'snacks' completely obsolete from your repertoire, as most models do, by simply eating the right amounts of proper food, so you won't ever need one. If you're caught out and need some energy, go for something with the guts to sustain you, such as a banana, or a packet of unroasted nuts, a small piece of cheese, an avocado or a hard-boiled egg. Something satisfying.

Frankly, juices don't hit the mark, nor does a low-fat biscuit, or raw vegetables with a dip. Can you imagine anyone but a lifestyle gurusome opening the fridge door and saying 'Wow, a carrot stick dipped in fat-free yoghurt, I can't wait.' Because they're there you'll eat the whole pack of biscuits, and you certainly won't be satisfied with the carrot stick. But who, apart from Paul Newman, would want to shovel down eight hard-boiled eggs in succession? The best foods to keep you away from crappy snacks (and you know what they are) contain both protein and fat.

'Health' drinks

All models know that canned, fizzy drinks are sugar hand grenades and that the 'diet' alternatives contain aspartame, which increases your desire to eat junk food. But they're also wary of the cunning calories hidden in many of the so-called 'health' drinks. There's a plethora of drinks with added herbal extracts, vitamins and minerals, which are blatantly marketed as wholesome. Let's take a typical well-known brand that boasts nine vitamins and 20 per cent fruit and has a convincingly healthy-looking label. The truth is the 500ml (17fl oz) bottle packs in more than 50g (2oz) of sugars and 200 calories. Even if 20 per cent of this is fruit sugar from the fruit juice, it still leaves eight teaspoons of 'sugar' sugar, which you could get from an orange and still have 136 calories to play with.

Fruit sugar (fructose) is better for us than sugar because it's absorbed more slowly and gives a gentler blood-sugar rise, but both supply the same amount of calories. So well-known drinks 'with herbal extracts' and which 'restore natural balance' still have over 120 calories per 330ml (11fl oz).

Then there are the healthy-looking mineral waters with 'a touch of fruit'. There's actually no fruit at all – it's fruit flavouring, which means around five teaspoons of added sugar per bottle. Why waste your calories on sugary drinks? Do what models do and drink water instead.

Let's do lunch

The ideal lunch is protein based: tuna, prawns, fresh or smoked salmon, chicken, turkey, ham, beef, cheese, egg – not forgetting tofu, of course, and should also include a small amount of grains and some vegetables. A sandwich with more filling than bread is the perfect choice.

You're more likely to want to nap after a lunch that's high in carbohydrates, so it's wiser to choose a turkey sandwich, on wholemeal (whole-wheat) bread, rather than a bowl of pasta. High-fat lunches (cheeseburger with fries!) will make you even more tired.

Sandwiches are the first choice for people on the move. We buy billions a year, so why oh why is the perfect sandwich so hard to find? That over-processed monstrosity filled with second-rate ingredients, enveloped in a sticky sauce, kept 'fresh' by chemicals and made in a giant sandwich factory four days before the sell-by date on the pack is still the norm.

Instead, search out a succulent panini stuffed with

glorious tomatoes, sweet prosciutto and milky mozzarella. A decent deli or sandwich shop will specialise in a diverse, delicious selection of sandwiches made with freshly baked bread, and simple top-class ingredients. The better delis will make you a designer sandwich on the spot to suit your discerning palette.

> *'My favourite is the ham and cheese sandwich you can order from room service at Claridges. They use gorgeous, smelly Gruyere.'*
>
> *Erin O'Connor*

Most breads are naturally low in fat apart from speciality breads, such as focaccia. Wholemeal (whole wheat) and wholegrain add extra fibre and minerals, but if you've stuffed your flexible restraint ratio, go for a tartine (French term for anything on toast) open sandwich, or peel off the top layer of bread (you won't be able to do this with cheap, garage-forecourt offerings because the filling and bread will be tragically bonded together with age and/or chemicals).

Sushi is a nutritious option that is low in fat and rich in omega-3s, but make sure it's fresh, and go easy on the soy sauce. You can opt for a salad, but watch out. You may think you're being virtuous, but most salads in supermarkets and restaurants are swimming in fatty dressings; a salad with dressing could contain as many calories as a burger and French fries! Look for those with separate dressings or a deli that makes up a salad on the spot to your specifications. Avoid dressings that come in pouches attached to supermarket salads, they're made with cheap vegetable oil, taste completely different and aren't good for you. Instead, make a dressing at home and take it to work in a plastic bottle. Home-made is best and couldn't be easier.

How to make the perfect vinaigrette

30ml (2 tbsp) good white wine vinegar

5ml (1 tsp) grainy mustard

1.5ml (¼ tsp) sea salt

a twist of freshly ground pepper

2.5ml (½ tsp) caster (superfine) sugar

half a garlic clove, finely chopped (optional)

120ml (8 tbsp) good fruity extra virgin olive oil

METHOD

1. Put all the ingredients except the olive oil in a screw-top jar and shake to mix thoroughly.

2. Drizzle in the olive oil, mixing all the time until it emulsifies like mayonnaise.

3. Add a drizzle to the salad at the last moment; any earlier and the leaves will go limp.

Salad scores

BEAN SALAD A good choice if not doused in olive oil. Beans are high in protein, fibre and B vitamins. High in good carbs, they have a low glycaemic index, so you'll feel full for longer.

CAESAR SALAD Not a great choice, as it is laden with fat, thanks to the Parmesan cheese, creamy dressing and croutons.

COLESLAW The shredded carrot is a nutritional power-house, a great source of fibre, vitamins A and C, betacarotene and folic acid, but the benefits are depleted by adding mayo. Make your own with fat-free yoghurt mixed with a little mayo. Eat it with some protein, such as quiche, to make a satisfying lunch.

GREEK SALAD A pretty good choice, as the tomatoes are high in vitamins C and A, and feta cheese is full of calcium and vitamin B_{12}; but watch the cheese, because of its fat content. Add olives (they're low in calories) for bulk.

POTATO SALAD A good source of potassium, fibre and vitamin C; but the mayo, however, is its downfall. Make your own with whole, unpeeled potatoes to avoid losing the vitamin C content; add chopped spring onions (scallions) and mix in a no-fat yoghurt dressing instead of mayo. Have it with some ham carved directly off the bone.

RICE SALAD A good healthy option if made with brown or wild rice, and with prawns added. Full of fibre, protein, B vitamins, iron and essential fatty acids. Raw (bell) peppers are an excellent source of vitamins A and C.

TUNA AND SWEETCORN Not bad in nutritional value, but its downfall could come from the oil in the canned tuna. Check that the tuna is packed in brine or spring water, or go for salmon, which has a better source of omega-3 fatty acids, or prawns, which are low in fat, good for vitamin B_{12} and rich in vitamins A, E and D.

> **TIP**
> - Rather than buying a big bag of leaves when you make your own green salad, buy a couple of Little Gem (Bibb) lettuces. The heads are tightly packed so they haven't been sprayed with pesticides to stop them looking frayed at the edges. Add a few leaves of watercress, spinach, parsley or radicchio.
> - When cut, soft herbs, such as chives, parsley and mint, begin to look tired; don't throw them away but revive them in a bowl of warm water for one minute. They suddenly get a new lease of live and return to their former selves.

Taking tea

You're more likely to catch a supermodel taking tea in a smart hotel with friends these days than swigging cocktails at the bar. We're not talking towers of cakes and trays of scones at the Ritz. That's tea for tourists. We're talking event tea, couture tea, which Elle Macpherson is partial to (herbal), as are Kate Moss and Naomi Campbell.

There are six main types of tea: black, green, white, oolong, scented and compressed. The most superior teas are grown at altitudes of 900–1,800m (3,000–6,000ft) above sea level, and Darjeeling, grown in the Himalayas, is the 'champagne of teas' and a supermodel favourite. Lapsang souchong from China, with its own, distinctive aroma, and Earl Grey, a mixture of Indian and China tea flavoured with bergamot oil, are also super-popular with models. Their brewing times are all-important. Darjeeling requires three to five minutes, Kenya from two to four and Chinese tea, five to seven minutes.

It's incredible how good tea is for you. It's credited with lowering blood pressure, helping prevent cancer and osteoporosis, lowering the risk of heart attack, helping prevent sun damage, being anti-viral, anti-inflammatory and anti-allergy, while new research reveals that drinking up to three cups a day of tea boosts your immune system and strengthens bones. It also helps to protect against tooth decay, and the facceine it contains make us feel alert and helps our concentration. Even regular tea bags are good for you, because black tea is naturally rich in flavonoids, protective antioxidants, whose levels rise significantly in the blood within 30–50 minutes of drinking a cup, although this effect is neutralised by adding milk.

> **TIP** It's best to eat iron-rich foods such as dark green leafy vegetables separately from drinking tea, as the tannin in tea reduces the ability of the body to absorb iron.

Both green tea and black tea come from the leaves of the plant *Camellia sinensis*, but the processing is different. Leaves for black tea are fully oxidised, while those for green teas are lightly steamed before being dried. Black teas come mostly from plantations in Africa, India, Sri Lanka and

Indonesia, while green teas come from countries in the Far East, such as China and Japan.

HERBAL TEAS have great soothing properties. The calming effect of camomile, traditionally a bedtime drink, can be enjoyed at any time of day to de-stress. Like peppermint tea, it also relaxes muscles and is good for alleviating menstrual cramps. Peppermint tea is a natural remedy for indigestion and can ease migraine and relieve the airways of asthma sufferers.

GREEN TEA is the supermodels' all-time favourite. It contains supernutrients called satechins that help the liver break down fat. This, combined with their ability to boost the metabolism, suggests green tea may help weight loss. A super-flavonoid, EGCG is more powerful an antioxidant than vitamin C and also has anti-cancer properties by blocking the body's production of the urokinase enzyme that cancer cells need to grow.

Green tea also provides a rare dietary source of vitamin K, which is important for building strong bones. You can drink any amount of green tea a day, but don't drink it at bedtime as one cup contains 40mg of caffeine. Milk neutralises the effect of the antioxidants.

Decaffeinated tea of any kind has less than 3mg of caffeine compared to the 40–60mg of standard tea. Yet it still retains its flavonoids, the main protective antioxidants associated with reducing heart disease and stroke, so is a good choice.

The perfect mint tea

Warm the teapot and add 2 teaspoons of green tea and 5 tablespoons of mint (spearmint is best). Boil the water, add it to the pot and leave to stand for five minutes. Pour the tea through a strainer into warmed glasses or small cups and add a little sugar, if you like it the Moroccan way.

Dinner tricks

Having dinner in a restaurant with friends is one of life's great pleasures. Variety *is* the spice of life, and discovering new tastes, or choosing old favourites which you can't be bothered to make at home, is a wonderfully, satisfying experience.

Great cooking has a transforming effect, bringing a mystical sense of well-being, and is a genuinely mind-altering experience. Furthermore, spicy foods produce endorphins, which lift your mood.

'I'm a big lover of good food; I particularly love pasta and cheese, and I really enjoy that whole thing of eating and drinking with friends. But I guess I don't eat too much of these, because I don't put on weight. Moderation is the key. Eat enough of your favourite foods to enjoy the delicious taste, but don't overdo it.'

Helena Christensen

Restaurant food usually has a high hidden calorie, fats and salt count. If your meal out is a treat, use your 80/20 flexible restraint rule and thoroughly enjoy it. At other times a meal is just a meal in a toxic environment and you have to use your skills to survive it. The key is to choose what you're eating rather than letting it choose you.

Chinese

LOVE IT

wonton soup

egg-drop soup

dim-sum steamed dumplings

stir-fried prawn, chicken, beef or vegetables

extra portion of steamed vegetables

boiled rice

fresh lychees

SKIP IT

sweet and sour chicken or pork – fatal!

beef with orange – no citrus in sight, just fried orange peel with breaded fried beef

food with cashew nuts – they're caramelised

spring rolls and prawn crackers

egg-fried rice

fruit fritters

Indian

LOVE IT

chicken/prawn/beef Madras

tandoori or tikka dishes (Indian kebabs)

SKIP IT

chicken/lamb korma – much too creamy

lamb, chicken or beef marsala – creamy

jalfrezi, rogan josh
  (tomato based)

chicken biryani – fried

Bombay potatoes

onion bhajis

gobi aloo saag

samosas

boiled rice and chapatis

bhajis, poppadoms, naan

Italian

LOVE IT

SKIP IT

Parma ham or bresaola
  with melon

antipasto – salamis and oily
  things

tricolore salad

spaghetti carbonara – creamy

chicken cacciatore

pizza

bowl of mussels

pasta primavera

pasta sauces: napolitana
  (tomato)

stuffed mushrooms

vongole (clams)

risotto

primavera(vegetables)

puttanesca (tomatoes,
  olives, vegetables)

zabaglione

Bolognese (meat)

seafood, chicken or meat
  'fritto'

fresh figs

cappuccino

If you're going **Greek**, choose a falafel sandwich or a
shish kebab, which has virtually no fat and is low in calories
because it's grilled; a doner kebab has twice the calories.
Thai food is a winner – it has lemongrass, coriander and
garlic, all great for bones and teeth, but watch the coconut.
Ditch the top of the bun with your **burger**, and if you're
eating **Tex-Mex** go for grilled fish, salads, chillies and rice or

a soft tortilla wrap rather than the sour cream, tortilla chips, deep-fried tortillas and mounds of guacamole.

Simply the best

I agree with gourmet Curnonsky's definition of good cooking: 'Things should taste of what they are.' Simple, fresh food, beautifully prepared and presented, using the best quality ingredients available, can't be beaten. It's also the true test of a great chef. What could be better on a hot summer's evening than the subtlest, sexiest asparagus, followed by golden-skinned, pearly breasted roast chicken, threaded with tarragon and eaten with sweet, nutty new potatoes and baby broad beans, no bigger than the nail on your little finger ... and a lightly chilled, perfectly chosen wine.

Not the house red

There's a new pill on the market that gives you all the benefits of red wine without having to drink it. How clever — none of the side effects of having to enjoy the taste! If you're living in the real world, here's the wise girl's guide to enjoying your wine.

Friends will be impressed with your new-found knowledge, but the real point is that cheap wine is like junk food: you're never, ever satisfied, however much you drink, and you feel lousy afterwards. A recent study of over 7,000 people, taken over a five-year period, showed that drinking up to three UK units of alcohol a day (a 125ml (4fl oz) glass of wine is one unit) had no effect on their weight. So the good news is that you can still enjoy the odd tipple and not feel guilty about piling on the pounds. Moderate doses relieve stress and relax the muscles – and the antioxidant polyphenols in red wine can help counteract the ageing process.

How to order wine

1. Don't go for the house wine unless you know it's good. Most aren't.

2. If you need one wine for a variety of dishes (fish, meat, vegetarian) go for a Pinot Noir, a Beaujolais Cru or a red Loire, such as Saumur-Champigny.

3. Familiar and easy-to-pronounce wines – Chablis, Sancerre, Cloudy Bay – will be less good value than a difficult to pronounce wine from an obscure region.

4. Avoid cheap, common Italian wines – Pinot Grigio, Frascati, Soave, Valpolicella – and take a chance on an unknown recent vintage from the south of Italy.

5. Australian dry Riesling is better value and more versatile with food than Chardonnay. It also ages well, unlike most other Aussie whites.

6. With all other New World whites, especially Sauvignon blanc, choose the youngest vintage available.

7. South African Sauvignon blancs are the new, often cheaper alternative to Sancerre, Pouilly Fume and New Zealand Sauvignon.

8. Except on their home territory, Californian wines are usually expensive compared to the same quality from the southern hemisphere.

9. Chilean and Argentinian reds can make a good inexpensive choice in place of Merlot and Cabernet Sauvignon.

10. Bordeaux is seldom a good buy, with high mark-ups and too many of the lesser vintages.

11. Burgundy is also expensive, but bargains (red and white) can be found among the less well-known villages and among domaine-bottled white Macons.

Best with

Chinese food: Riesling or demi-sec champagnes
Thai: Sauvignon blanc or a New World dry Riesling
Japanese: German Riesling and brut champagnes
Indian: unoaked Semillion or Riesling, Gewürztraminer for highly spiced dishes

---

Sham pain

We all know that turning wine into a **spritzer** with sparkling water halves the calories by making the wine last longer, but the clever bit is that it hydrates you while it dehydrates you! If it's serious bubbles you're after then a **Buck's Fizz** with its three-to-one mix of bubbles and orange juice has only about 77 calories per glass, plus the added bonus of a shot of vitamin C, which will help ward off a hangover.

> **TIP** Look out for the supermodels' favourite tipple: Laurent Perrier Ultra Brut Champagne. Normal champagne comes in at about 95 calories per glass, but the smart model choice, having fermented away all its sugar, slips in with just 60 calories a glass.

If bubbles don't hit the mark then try a **North Pole** – dry vermouth topped with pineapple juice – or a **Seabreeze** of cranberry juice with vodka and grapefruit juice, both clocking in at 180 calories (the juice technically counts toward your 'five pieces of fruit and vegetables a day' quota. Stay away from alcopops – the highest in calories. As if!

> *'My favourite room-service drink is champagne. It's very convenient. You can have it for breakfast, in a cocktail, at lunchtime, with a sandwich and all night long.'*
>
> *Erin O'Connor*

Flying

Standard airline food is crap, and models, who travel constantly, know to ring the airline ahead and order a special menu. Although airlines tend not to make this public knowledge, they're quite happy to offer you a wide range of low fat, low calorie, low cholesterol, kosher, vegetarian and other choices. Different airlines have different criteria to define these different meals, and you may find the vegetarian option is almost invariably higher in fat than other choices as it's usually based on cheese. The low-calorie meals are probably better to order than the low-fat meals as the low-fat meals often turn out to be high in cholesterol, which still has an overall high fat content. The low-calorie options tend to be better meals all round.

On short-haul trips models pack their own goody bags – unsalted freeze-dried nuts, a banana or apple, a couple of hard-boiled eggs and the ubiquitous bottle of mineral water. They also make sure their last meal before setting out has a good balance of protein and starch, so that they feel motivated and satisfied, rather than lethargic.

For a long-haul flight, fill a 2-litre (3½ pint) bottle of mineral water with a sachet of multivitamin powder, set your watch for the time of your destination and don't even think about alcohol. Take a tip from Helena Christensen and spritz water on your face. Helena's favourite is Remo Facial mist, which she picks up at Sydney's most fashionable store of the same name, but other models swear by Evian or Vichy sprays.

Celebrations
....

Your birthday, Christmas Day, Thanksgiving – go on, live it up. They only happen once a year. A big blowout isn't what spells trouble; it's eating too much the days before and after that do the damage. Avoid crossing the line by keeping active and going for long, brisk walks. Roast turkey with lots of vegetables is one of the healthiest meals around. If you stick to basics, avoid lashings of bread sauce, piles of stuffing and second helpings of roast potatoes, you'll come out unscathed. Try these:

- Sit opposite a mirror when you eat. You eat less when you catch sight of your reflection.

- Wear Bridget Jones knickers. When they start digging in, you'll know to stop pigging out.

- Turn up the lights. Dim lighting reduces inhibitions around food, so you eat more.

Pre-party planning

- Drink plenty of water before setting off.

- Eat something bulky, such as bread and a banana (potassium fortifies the liver).

- Have a glass of milk, a smoothie or a yoghurt to line your stomach.

- If you know in advance it's going to be a real head-banger, take 500mg of GLA (gamma linoleic acid, the main ingredient in evening primrose oil), 1g of vitamin C, a B complex, plus a milk thistle supplement with a full glass of water before you go out.

At the party

- Alternate one glass of alcohol with one glass of water.

- Don't mix grain and grape.

- Don't mix the mixers – it's hard for the body.

- Avoid fruit-based drinks – the sweetness disguises the amount of alcohol.

Before bed

Eat three pieces of fruit when you get home and one piece every time you get up at night; it combats damage by free radicals. Or drink a vanilla bean and honey smoothie, which contains stomach-soothing probiotics, or a fruit-based smoothie.

Rules for when you're out and about

....

1. If you're always too rushed for breakfast, get everything ready the night before. Eat breakfast every day, and include at least one serving of fruit.

2. Only reach for a snack if you're genuinely hungry, and make sure it's got guts and is a complete food (banana, nuts, and so on), not a man-made 'snack'.

3. Have protein and two servings of vegetables for lunch.

4. Don't let the size of the serving put down in front of you determine how much you eat. Stop eating when you're satisfied.

5. Drink at least 1 litre (1¾ pints) of water throughout the day, and turn your back on fizzy, 'diet', 'sports', 'energy' and 'health' drinks. They'll disrupt your new energy levels.

6. Don't waste calories nibbling bread before the meal arrives. Fizzy mineral water will fill the gap.

7. If you really want the bread, swap the butter for olive oil. You'll eat less because the oil feels richer in your mouth.

8. Order dressings separately and drizzle them on sparingly. Don't pour on a sauce, dip your fork in it.

9. Allow 20 minutes per course – the time your body needs to send satiety signals. If you feel full, stop ordering.

10. Don't give yourself excuses to eat bad food. If you find yourself in a mediocre restaurant or hotel, order food that has to be cooked on the spot, and is therefore totally fresh, such as an omelette or grilled meat and a salad you can dress yourself.

11. Eat four times more vegetables and salad to protein (meat, fish, eggs, cheese) or carbohydrate (rice, pulses, bread, potatoes).

12. It's not as hard as it looks to eat five portions of fruit and vegetables every day – fresh, frozen or dried. A glass of juice for breakfast, a large bowl of salad for lunch followed by a piece of fruit and two vegetables with dinner.

13. If you eat more wholegrain carbohydrate food you will automatically reduce your intake of fat.

14. Quash sugar cravings with chromium-rich foods, such as shellfish and cheese, and wholemeal products, such as wholemeal (whole-wheat) bread, cereals and pastas. Protein-packed foods, such as chicken, fish, eggs, pulses, lentils and lean red meat, also ward off sugar urges.

> **TIP** Carry a small bottle of vanilla essence in your bag and take a sniff, or rub it on the back of your hand every time you feel a sugar craving coming on.

15. Choose strong, vibrant-tasting food so that you don't feel deprived; fish, prawns and chicken, with chilli, garlic or herbs, such as coriander (cilantro) and basil, are good choices.

16. Learn to recognise food with quality and freshness. If you don't recognise its provenance and what's in it (a hot dog?), don't eat it.

17. Stick to fruit-based puddings, such as baked apples, poached pears, or, best of all, choose berries (blueberries, raspberries, strawberries, blackberries).

18. Have a maximum of four cups of coffee or tea a day, except for herbal or decaffeinated. Don't have milk in tea. Both green and black tea contains antioxidants, but their effect is neutralised by adding milk.

19. Remember to eat regular meals. It balances blood sugars, reduces food cravings, optimises metabolic rate (at which calories are burned) and leads to healthy weight control.

20. Remember: a little of what you fancy does you good. What's the point in living longer and being thinner, if you don't enjoy life?

11

How models balance exercise and diet

Helena Christensen doesn't have one; Elle Macpherson and Claudia Schiffer do. Strict workout regimes suit some supermodels and not others, confirming my theory that the world is divided into those who enjoy exercise and those who prefer to watch them.

> *'I've always enjoyed a varied workout, combining power-walking with yoga'*
> **Claudia Schiffer**

Helena's less rigid approach doesn't mean her body isn't up to scratch. In fact, she has the body most other models say they envy most, but she chooses to bypass rigorous workouts, while still adhering to the non-negotiable rule – that the only way to maintain a slim figure is by eating an amount of food in direct proportion to what your body can burn off. How you stick to this rule is as individual and personal to you as your DNA. But one thing is for sure: you won't keep your body fit and slim if you don't find a satisfactory, enjoyable method of burning off what you eat. The world is littered with unused gym memberships and unloved leotards.

> *'I went to a British school (Gordonstoun), which was somewhat inclined towards tough sports. I was quite a lunatic in my youth and loved mountain-parachuting and bungee jumping. Now I'm hooked on marathon running, which I do to raise money for animal charities. I find it enormously gratifying to push myself to the very edge.'*
>
> *India Hicks*

The way forward is to weigh up your options realistically. If your job entails dashing around and using heaps of energy, you obviously need less exercise than if you sit around an office all day. And if you regularly go clubbing and dancing in the evening, you don't need as much exercise as when your hobby is reading.

TIP Exercising outside burns 12 per cent more calories than the same workout indoors, as the body burns more to keep warm. In summer you burn even more through sweating.

If you've joined a gym because you feel a bit guilty after a Christmas blowout, you won't stay the course if it makes you feel bored, guilty, pressurised or resentful, however much you think you will. Convincing excuses will somehow pop into your head, forcing you to miss session after session. This is because your subconscious mind doesn't think of the form of exercise you've chosen as fun and a positive experience, so it sabotages your conscious attempts to get to the gym, making it very difficult to motivate yourself. Sticking with exercise is as much to do with your head as your body.

If I speak with confidence, it's because I know about this stuff. Ever since I won a cup for my school by winning a 100-yard sprint race, I've been so indelibly frozen in nostalgic shock and glory that I haven't run for anything since. The very word 'push-up' gives me the bends, and Ab Fab is something I prefer to watch than acquire. But I'm the same weight now as in my modelling days, so I must be doing something right.

Here's the deal: to lose 450g (1lb) of fat you need to burn about 3,500 calories. That's six hours of running on a treadmill (600 calories an hour), seven hours riding a bike (500 calories an hour) or eight to nine hours of fast walking (450 calories an hour). In food terms it's the equivalent of two large bowls of spaghetti carbonara, five bottles of wine and about ten chocolate bars.

If you had a chocolate bar every day beyond your body's calorie requirement, you would gain about 15kg (33lb) of fat within a year. However, if you walked fast for an hour a day, you could lose 23kg (52lb) in a year. It's simple: **if you like to eat and you don't exercise, you'll get fat.**

The female body needs around 1,900 calories a day to

maintain her weight comfortably. If you drastically reduce the amount you eat, you're in danger of slowing down your metabolic rate. But if you increase your activity rate, you will be burning unwanted fat reserves with gusto. The most effective way to create this good-energy deficit is to exercise consistently, but not too harshly, for 30 minutes a day at least five times a week, or for around four times a week for at least 40 minutes, with your exercise divided into these three parts:

1. Twenty minutes of any activity that increases your heart rate and causes you to consume more oxygen (aerobic) – fast walking, swimming, cycling, dancing, trampolining, table tennis.

2. Ten minutes of any type of exercise that isn't obviously aerobic and helps sculpt the body (anaerobic) – lifting weights, isometrics.

3. Ten minutes of stretching (callisthenics) – yoga, Pilates, tai chi.

If you're seriously 'going for it' and contemplating a Sophie Dahl type of transformation, then a truly focused fitness programme is essential with the help of a personal trainer, to make sure you're doing it right.

> **TIP** To burn more calories during a swim, spend 30 seconds treading water after every two lengths at the deep end. Keep your legs straight and your toes pointed.

For the rest of us mere mortals, the US Surgeon General recently declared that moderate activity for 30 minutes a day is *the* most effective way of controlling weight. Regular walking in 10–30-minute bouts actually burns more calories than doing one prolonged session, due to the effect of exercise on the metabolism. It not only elevates your metabolic rate while you're doing it but also keeps your calorie-burning meter cranked up for long periods after you finish. So you continue to burn calories even after you've stopped moving.

A daily brisk walk of 30 minutes could lead to 5.5kg (12lb) weight loss over a year. Walking keeps you alert, is a great antidote to depression and exercises every part of you. You can also do it anywhere, apart from Los Angeles where they make you join a gym.

If you complement this with core exercises to tone and improve your posture, and try to find time to fit more 'lifestyle' activity into your day, you need never, ever cross the threshold of a gym, do an aerobics class, don a leotard or run around a park.

TIP If your plans for the day mean you can't exercise all in one go, make sure you use the three-minutes-an-hour rule. Every hour get up and walk around for at least three minutes. That adds up to 30 minutes a day, the minimum for good health.

Those who go for the burn are also at risk from rewarding themselves for being active. They think they're burning off far more calories than they actually are. Even if you do 30 minutes in an exercise class or on equipment such as a treadmill or a bicycle, you're unlikely to work off more than 300 calories. Gym sessions should be the icing on the cake not the only activity you ever do.

> 'I like to ride my horses early in the morning. It's just me and my horses against the world. I play polo, which means I ride all the time. I play a lot of golf too. Both keep me pretty active, so I don't really feel as though I actually need to go to the gym.'
>
> **Jodie Kidd**

We often think we're more active than we really are. We may have been geographically or mentally active, sitting in a cab or train, but that's not physically active. Every night, check that you've physically moved your body for 30 minutes during the day. Always be active outside your exercise sessions and take on board that moderately paced, sustained activities, such as climbing the stairs, can promote weight loss more effectively than brief, high intensity workouts.

Truly lazy or just uninspired?

Motivation is the key to sticking with an exercise regime – and mine is Arthur (my dog), who takes me for a 30-minute walk, morning and evening, every day, come rain or shine. It's finally become a mutual pleasure, and the routine is now as familiar as brushing my teeth. Before Arthur, I used to do the housework with great gusto, to very loud music – Stevie Wonder worked best.

If you see walking as an isolated, tedious, repetitious kind of thing, but quite like the ease of it, get some head-phones, and listen to your newest CD or the latest thriller on tape. You'll have walked five blocks before you know it.

> *My dog and I run the entire length of the beach outside my house every morning, which is four miles long. It's at that moment that I feel "this is why I live on this island"— because I have a pink-sand beach at the bottom of my garden which I love to make good use of.'*
>
> *India Hicks*

If walking doesn't grab you at all, there are stacks of other 'why not' aerobic choices around. Fencing is popular with New York models, or you could try salsa dancing, rollerblading, skating, golf, tennis, horse-back riding, ping pong, boxing, trampolining, swimming ... and then there's sport. Whatever happened to sport?

> *I just love playing tennis. It's a really good workout. I play tennis with friends in the country every weekend.'*
>
> *Claudia Schiffer*

Netball, tennis and hockey have all been usurped by the solitary world of the treadmill. Exercising can be sociable, fun, skilful, graceful and challenging. It needn't be dull, self-punishing and lonely. Make enjoyment your aim, rather than some kind of perfect body image.

> **TIP** Ten minutes' bouncing on a trampoline gives you the same benefits as 30 minutes' jogging and is much better for your joints. Extra beneficial for thighs, it's the ultimate exercise for tackling cellulite, because rebounding strengthens the ligaments and tones all the major muscles and connective tissues.

Exercise for your state of mind

SHORT-TERM NERVES (JOB INTERVIEW/HOT DATE) High-energy exercise, such as jogging or boxercise.

ONGOING ANXIETY Slow-paced, relaxed activities, like Pilates. Take exercise with others to take the focus off yourself.

SHORT-TERM SADNESS (RELATIONSHIP BREAK-UP, REDUNDANCY) Participate in group activities; staring into the mirror will only make you feel worse.

LONGER-TERM SADNESS Find an up-beat instructor who understands the power of positive thinking. Swimming helps. Long-term depression needs long-term goals.

ANGER AND FRUSTRATION Interval training – high intensity, short bursts with short rests.

Walking tall, model style

Elizabeth Hurley looks positively Amazonian when she's 'on show' and arrives at a film premiere, and Kate Moss's legs appear to go on forever whenever she struts the catwalk, but both these girls are average height. By perfecting their posture they give the illusion of being 3kg (7lb) lighter and several inches taller instantly. Constantly posing for photographs teaches them how to set their bodies for the camera in order to make a total impact. Standing upright with their shoulders relaxed and their upper body face on to the world, they send out strong messages that they're powerful and confident.

Although posture is partly genetic, most people automatically slouch when they sit or walk. The trick to having a great figure is not just standing up straight – it's being strong enough to stay up there without thinking. Most people with poor posture agree that when they finally do stand or sit properly, it gets tiring after a few minutes. That's because the muscles aren't used to being held this way, so you need to retrain and strengthen them.

Three ways to stand taller

1. If you work sitting at a desk all day, try folding a small cushion into a hard wedge, then put this in the middle of your chair and sit on the edge of it. This will tilt your pelvis forward and down, forcing your spine to sit perfectly upright.

2. Sit on the edge of your chair. You'll notice that your back straightens instantly. If you sit like this for a few hours every day, your body will slowly get used to being in that position, so you'll stand and walk with much better posture all the time.

3. Turn your knees out very slightly when you walk or run, even if you exaggerate a bit at first to get used to the feeling. Over time this will eventually shorten the buttock muscles so they lift and appear ultra-toned.

Fitness videos

These haven't changed much in the 20 years since Jane Fonda launched her mega-selling *Workout* video. Cindy Crawford, Elle Macpherson and Claudia Schiffer have all since produced less fierce fitness videos than the Fonda 'high impact' version, which involved constant pounding of the joints and going for the 'burn'; this has proved to be bad news for the body long term, often destroying cartilage that protects the joints.

The real problem is that most people who buy exercise videos never do more than watch them, because the videos aren't inclusive enough. There's no time for explanation, correction or individual instructions and they all feature fast-paced, cardio-based routines that require a good deal of flexibility. However, videos can be a good introduction to yoga and Pilates, with their emphasis on teaching basic techniques and skills, such as good posture and breathing, core stability and stretching. All these are key to building what is known as muscle memory, the basic know-how essential for successful toning and shaping, before moving on to more active physical pursuits.

Three great gadgets to get you fit

Find these inexpensive gizmos, or similar, from good sports shops worldwide:

BALANCE BOARD If you haven't got time for Pilates lessons, this 40cm (16in) wobble board is a good compromise. The aim is to balance on the board so that neither edge touches the floor. Good fun.

PEDOMETER A battery-operated credit-card-size device you clip on to your clothing to record every step you take. The good old US Surgeon General recommends aiming for 10,000 steps a day to stay fit.

CALORIE JUMP Skipping is a great all-round exercise that will help burn fat, strengthen bones and tone muscles. This lightweight rope counts the number of skips you take and calculates the number of calories burned (10 minutes to burn a slice of fruit cake).

TIP Don't 'treat yourself' for completing your exercises, as many fitness experts and coaches advocate. Your mind will think it's being rewarded for coping with a 'difficult task' when moving your body about is what it's designed to do.

Not a fat chance

Walking

- Uses all the major muscle groups if you swing your arms with each step

- Burns as many calories as jogging the same distance

- Distance is more important than speed

- Can be done anytime, anywhere

Exercise bike

- Works the major low muscle groups without stress on knees or back

- Strengthens the muscles in preparation for brisk walking and jogging

- Cardiovascular and respiratory benefits

Swimming

- Involves all the major muscle groups

- Cardiovascular fitness without stressing joints

Pilates

- Strengthens core muscles, creating a firm base for other exercise

- Restores strength to the stomach muscles without sit-up stress

- Excellent for the very obese

- Easy to learn – you don't have to do regular exercise

Ten reality checks

1. Stop kidding yourself that celebrities have some secret that you don't.

2. Stop pretending you don't have time.

3. Take responsibility for your body.

4. Set aside a regular time for exercise.

5. Be realistic, you're not going to run every morning.

6. Only go to the gym if you really want to.

7. Realise 'you' are not fat, but your choices have led to a body that is.

8. You'll never reach your destination if you don't know where you're going.

9. Find a healthy project that gets you so excited you can't wait to start.

10. Make sure you walk briskly, or do some similar moderately intense activity for 30 minutes on at least five days a week.

12

Summary for success

Any change in behaviour feels exciting for the first few days – a positive new step – but during the second week, our established habits, the ones we're comfortable with, try to click back into play and our resolve wavers. The ups and downs of daily life sometimes make coping with change hard. But we're living in the real world where there will always be stress, and food can't resolve stressful situations. It won't repair relationships. It won't settle arguments.

Most negative feelings are created and dominated by being overtired. Tiredness can make everything look bleak, but learning to stand back and recognising that it is not reality, just a physical passing moment, is the secret to staying on track.

Eating and sleeping will feed your nervous system and your psyche. Getting at least five hours of good solid sleep helps to balance your levels of the fat-storing hormone, insulin, so you can be slim while you snore.

TIP Learn to enjoy your own company. For 10 minutes every day, whisk yourself to a quiet place and concentrate on your own thoughts; think, reassess and stabilise. Focus on what's really important to you, and act on it. A daily mini-meditation will bring the benefit of centring you, and with that comes balance.

Eight tips for a good night's sleep

1. Avoid caffeine after 4.00 p.m. and silly quantities of alcohol.

2. Avoid pork, bacon, cheese, chocolate, aubergines (eggplant), tomatoes, potatoes and wine near bedtime as they're rich in tyramine, an amino acid the body can convert into noradrenalin, a brain stimulant.

3. Avoid high-sugar foods, they're an instant source of energy at the wrong time.

4. Avoid aspartame sweetener; it's a stimulant that depletes sleep-promoting chemicals in the blood.

5. Avoid spicy foods and hot spices, as these act as stimulants.

6. Avoid processed food, as it stresses the liver.

7. Avoid no food – stressful to the whole body.

8. Boost your serotonin levels by eating foods rich in tryptophan, which induces sleepiness, by having:

   a) a small pot of natural yoghurt with sunflower seeds, chopped dates or figs and banana, or

   b) a banana milkshake (with cow's milk or soya), or

   c) fruit and sunflower seeds/almonds, or

   d) dried dates and sunflower seeds/almonds.

'Getting the right amount of sleep every night would have to be my best secret. I look better, feel better, and seem to radiate more happiness when I've had lots of sleep.'

Catherine Hurley

Don't let PMS sabotage your new regime

Changes in hormone levels can trigger a desire for high-cal, high-carb foods, which increase in intensity until your period begins. Certain foods minimise these fluctuations, keeping blood-sugar levels steady, beating cravings and helping control high levels of oestrogen.

■ Eat lighter foods that are low in protein in the days leading up to your period because heavy demands on your digestive system will drain your energy and divert oxygen from your brain. Eat plenty of fish and vegetables, fruit for glucose, and avoid alcohol and caffeine – they make you jittery and irritable.

- Avoid salty food, as salt leads to water retention and makes you feel bloated.

- Try to cook your food from scratch whenever possible during this time and avoid adding salt to meals.

- Don't believe that the less water you drink, the less fluid your body retains. The opposite is true. If you suffer from water retention it's because you don't drink enough. If you restrict fluids, your body will try to compensate by retaining liquid.

- Food containing magnesium helps to reduce pains, by easing uterine muscle contractions, especially when taken with calcium.

- Stay clear of sugary foods. They release more insulin into your body, which is converted into fat, causing your body to fail to break down previously stored fat. Your higher weight then increases oestrogen production and creates a hormone imbalance, resulting in further sugar cravings.

- Eating plenty of fibre prevents food from putrefying inside your body causing it to bloat. It also helps digestion, increases your feeling of fullness and removes toxins from your body.

- Once your period has started, drink lots of water and herbal teas, and balance the lower protein intake of the past few days with plenty of easily digestible protein, such as chicken soup. Avoid fatty foods and very cold foods, which can cause spasms in the uterus.

The role of vitamins and minerals

Eating fresh, organic local produce from all the food groups – and avoiding additives, preservatives, pesticides and hydrogenated fat, as much as possible – results in super-models needing to take very few supplements.

During times of high pressure, often when the major designers show their collections and models make endless quick, backstage changes in several shows a day, the girls will take a top-quality multivitamin and mineral as an insurance policy. However, they never, ever buy cheap brands of vitamins and minerals, as they know that they're completely useless. The supplement models regularly favour is Berocca, a high-dose formulation of essential vitamins and minerals, in the form of a lozenge added to water, which makes a delicious, effervescent, tropical-tasting drink. It contains 1,000mg of vitamin C plus B complex and zinc, making it the perfect skin repairer and immunity booster. Models take Berocca because they know our bodies don't manufacture vitamin C, and as it's water soluble, we excrete it every three or four hours. Vitamin C hates being stored, so it's possible a supplement has a higher nutrient level than fresh oranges on shelves, picked weeks ago, and ripened in transit.

Vitamin facts

■ Nutrients work as a team. If you take mega doses of one, it can block the absorption of another. High doses of zinc block the absorption of iron, for example.

- It's best to take vitamins just before meals so that they mix with food in the stomach and are more easily absorbed.

- Don't take supplements with tea or coffee, as those drinks block the absorption of a range of vitamins. Any hot drink will kill the good bacteria in a probiotic supplement if drunk within 30 minutes of taking.

- If you're anaemic and are taking iron supplements, take them with vitamin C rich foods, which enhance absorption. Do not take them with wheat, fizzy drinks or antacid medications, all of which stop iron entering the blood.

- Some 'super-mega' types of vitamins do more harm than good. Excessive quantities of vitamin B_6 alone can lead to peripheral neuropathy (loss of feeling in your arms and legs).

- Don't buy cheap vitamins. There are no patents on the manufacture of vitamins and anyone can jump on the bandwagon and market cheap pills, which do you no good at all. Stick to ones that provide around 100 per cent of the recommended daily allowance (RDA).

- Never swig back vitamin pills with an alcoholic drink, as virtually none of the contents will be absorbed.

- Of the major vitamins, some are water-soluble, and some are oil-soluble. Water-solubles must be taken into the body daily, as they cannot be stored. These include vitamins C and B-complex.

■ Oil-soluble vitamins can be stored for longer periods in the body's fatty tissue and liver, and can cause tissue or organ damage if too much is taken. These include vitamins A, D, E and K.

Natural vitamins for glowing skin

Fruit, especially berries, boosts your vitamin C intake. It contains the supernutrient anthocyanidin, which strengthens the tiny blood vessels that deliver nutrients and oxygen to the skin.

Brazil nuts are the richest source of selenium, needed to help protect the natural moisturising oils present in the skin's upper layers.

Keeping it simple

....

While reading this book you may have noticed that, contrary to most diet books, I don't suggest you write lists, do calorie counts, check the GI (glycaemic index) of the food you eat, or say affirmations. This is because I figure you know all about that stuff. This is not the first 'diet' book you've read, and you don't need to write lists, because you're not stupid. You know instinctively that a slice of Black Forest gâteau will make you fatter than an orange, and you know whether you ate it or not.

The simple supermodel message is that if you give your body fewer empty calories, and provide it with more nutrient-dense alternatives, logically it will be satisfied sooner and require less food. Cut out the junk and don't snack – but if you have to, do it with protein/fat foods because they're basically self-limiting. Everyone's eaten a packet of biscuits at one go, but it's pretty difficult to eat ten hard-boiled eggs.

Wait until you're hungry before eating, drink water instead of fizzy drinks, override your penchant for second helpings, replace sugary things with ripe fruit, and learn to love and appreciate food that's good for you.

'Getting it'

You'll never succeed if you can't get past the notion that a diet is something you get on and then off, like a bus. If you can't get your head straight about food and weight, this book won't help. You have simply to 'get it'. Get the point of it. See that it makes sense. Your motivations will suddenly become clear and powerful; your self-esteem and your belief in your ability will be different this time. 'Getting it' will either dawn on you slowly, or hit you like turning on a light switch. You'll know when it happens.

Taking responsibility

The fast-food industry has a lot to answer for, constantly capitalising on its knowledge that the sugar/fat combination in snacks and fast foods can be virtually addictive. But the therapeutic culture we live in encourages us to shirk our own responsibilities, and not hold ourselves to account for our failings. Someone else is always to blame. Isn't it time we were honest with ourselves and admitted that our weaknesses are just that: bad habits that we can overcome if we really want to. We're not spoiled children devoid of any responsibility for our lives. We're grown adults capable of taking decisions. If you eat too many burgers, the chain you buy them from are not to blame. They don't exactly shovel it down your throat. You made the choice.

Staying on the straight and narrow

The supermodels' diet regime is about self-maintenance, not self-obsession. It's not about striving to reach some mythical goal in an endless daily struggle. It is about following the model rules of 'flexible restraint' where you eat healthy delicious food for 80 per cent of the time and treat yourself for the remainder. Staying in shape isn't about cutting certain food groups out of your life, but about eating food that you enjoy, that truly satisfies you psychologically, as well as physically filling you.

It doesn't take superhuman willpower to change your ways, only the wisdom to put yourself into a position where you don't need it. Choosing your food rather than letting it choose you will become a natural part of your life within six weeks of reading this book. That's how long it takes for a new pattern of behaviour to become a habit.

When you begin to eat the nutrients your body and brain need to produce serotonin, your taste for food will change, and you'll no longer crave nutritionally deficient food. Your taste automatically changes in about nine days, when healthy, wholesome foods actually start to taste better. The feedback you get from your body then makes it easy to stay on track.

Having realistic expectations

You may never be your perfect size 8, but you can make your body the best body you've ever had, if you don't fall into the trap of demanding a weight-loss schedule and perfect figure that exists only in your head. That we should judge one another by appearance is not a new phenomenon, but seldom have we been so immersed in a culture in which the much-touted 'ideal' physical shape for a woman is so ridiculously bizarre. A skeletal pre-pubescent boy's body with a large lollipop head, and the ever-present, paid-for cleavage is not the perfect body. And even the perfect body does not guarantee a perfect life. Hollywood is littered with sad, desperate women working out in their personal gyms, and shrinking their bodies to achieve more empty space to get lonelier in.

Scientists believe that ten years from now, the Western world will have morphed into two distinct body shapes: very thin or obese. It's already happening in America. So I have an outlandish idea: why don't those of us who are truly intrepid, decide to go out on a limb, be really unusual, break the rules – and aim to be normal. It's the post-modern way to be different.

Hugh Grant is one of our favourite customers at the deli, but it's Colin Firth who spoke these words of wisdom:

'When I made the first *Bridget Jones* film I was amazed that Renée Zelwegger was considered "fat" in the film. She didn't look fat to me as Bridget Jones — not at all. It didn't even occur to me that she was in any way overweight. There's all this self-torture thing going on. It's not attractive, it's not healthy, and it's not sexy.'

How true, Mr Darcy, how true.

Because you're worth it

You deserve to feel and look good, to enjoy the happiness, health and a sense of well-being that goes hand in hand with a fabulous, sensible and realistic diet. Then another thing will happen. A new feeling will wash over you in waves, in a way you've never experienced before. It will open doors for you, move mountains for you, make you respected and valued beyond your wildest dreams. It's called confidence – self-confidence. Once you really have it, you'll never underestimate its power.

'A designer said to me at a fitting "These trousers are a bit snug", so I replied, "Well, make the trousers bigger then." You have to stand up for yourself and have confidence. I'm glad I made a stand.'

Erin O'Connor

For mail-order details of the unusual or unique food products discussed in this book, and for delicious 'one-pot' recipes, log on to www.supermodelssecrets.com or to discover more about the author log on to www.victorianixon.com.

Index